Mindfulness for Seniors

A Flexible Wisdom-Driven Approach for
Revealing Joy & Meeting Life's Challenges

Blair O'Neil

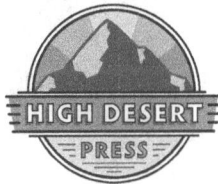

Mindfulness for Seniors

A Flexible Wisdom-Driven Approach for Revealing Joy & Meeting Life's Challenges

First Edition Printing ©2025 - High Desert Press / Blair & Jenna O'Neil
— All Rights Reserved —

ISBN 979-8-9992774-0-4 (Paperback)

Disclaimer: The author is not a medical or mental health professional. The content of this book is provided for informational and educational purposes only and is not intended as a substitute for professional medical advice, diagnosis, or treatment. While mindfulness offers valuable tools for well-being, it is not a substitute for professional medical, therapeutic, or emotional intervention.

We understand the unique challenges seniors may face. Readers are strongly encouraged to consult with their physician or other qualified healthcare provider with any questions they may have regarding a medical condition or before making any changes to their healthcare regimen or adopting any techniques or strategies described in this book. Never disregard professional medical advice or delay in seeking it because of something you have read in this book.

Our approach to mindfulness is designed to complement, not replace, existing medical and support services. Any application of the material set forth in this book is at the reader's discretion and sole responsibility. No specific outcomes are guaranteed. The author and publisher assume no liability for any injuries or damages that may result from the use of information contained within this book.

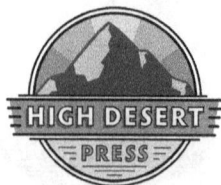

HighDesertPress.com

Reno, NV

Dedication:

To my wife, Jenna, for her patience while I created the entirety of the Mindfulness for Seniors project, including this book. Despite my long hours and notable lack of availability, she has been supportive every step of the way.

Acknowledgment:

I wish to acknowledge the lifetime of countless contributions of my family, friends, advisors, professional co-workers, clients, as well as my spiritual family and teachers, both living and those now departed, who freely shared their gifts and wisdom, and also presented me with the challenges that forged the person I am today. For each of their contributions I am forever grateful. It is my hope that their gifts have contributed to this book's usefulness and relevance for helping to ease the challenges of each reader as well as enhance their capacity for joy.

Table Of Contents

Introduction Part One: Getting Oriented:

Introduction Part Two: Core Concepts:

Introduction Part Three:
Obstacles, Misconceptions & History:

Foundations of Practical Mindfulness:

Core Mindfulness Exercises:

Mindfulness For All of Life:

Back Matter:

Intro Section 1

"The river of mindfulness
is beautiful and wide
and you can enter
any place you choose..."

From "Mindfulness for Seniors"

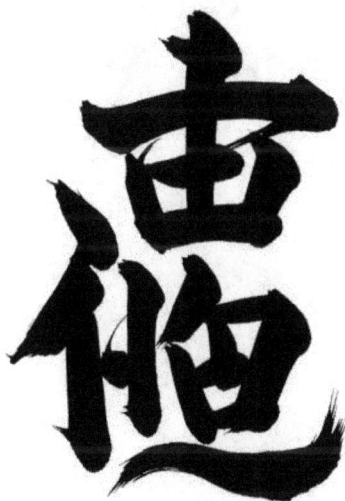

Getting Oriented

TABLE OF CONTENTS for

INTRODUCTION PART ONE: GETTING ORIENTED

Introduction Part One: Getting Oriented

"Start where you are.
Use what you have. Do what you can."

- Author Ashe
(Tennis Legend and Humanitarian)

I. A Unique Approach to Mindfulness

A Simple & Adaptable Wisdom-Driven Life Tool for Seniors

The river of mindfulness is beautiful and wide and you can enter any place you choose... so don't overthink it... just go with what resonates for you!

As for this book, it isn't just another guide to mindfulness. It offers a distinct path—a road less traveled, layered over the foundations of traditional mindfulness. A path where we invite you to explore a more relaxed, flexible, and open approach, an approach that we believe, while suitable for anyone, provides significant real-world benefits for seniors.

The path I share in this book fully embraces the big and small life challenges... It's an approach built not just on my own journey, but on the wisdom generously shared by my family, friends, and teachers over many years. An approach that also encourages the savoring and appreciating life's joys, instead of being simply focusing on problems or difficulities that must be solved. The approach is inclusive, gentle, and easy to try and understand.

As a fellow senior, I understand and appreciate the myriad changes and challenges that punctuate these later years of life—from health issues to the loss of loved ones and redefining our purpose in retirement and beyond.

Through a lens inspired by the rich wisdom traditions of Dzogchen and Vajrayana, and tempered by my life's journey, I offer a friendly, encouraging, down-to-earth, and non-spiritual approach, free from the jargon, clinician-speak, and prescriptive, goal-oriented approaches that are found in so many of the well-known mindfulness methodologies.

The essence of my approach is this: to create a practical, accessible, flexible, and easy-to-use Mindfulness Toolkit for meeting life head-on in all its myriad forms, both the joys and sorrows. It's an accommodating and direct invitation that we believe cuts to the heart of the matter, starting with a **"micro-mindfulness moments"** approach, recognizing that even a single mindful breath has the potential to radically transform our perception, and moves to slightly longer exercise options, and finally to the extended deep relaxation techniques.

To truly grasp our unique perspective, let's explore the key aspects of our approach and how they differ from other mindfulness perspectives and methods:

Key Aspects of This Approach:

• **Open, Spacious Awareness (Beyond "Doing"):**
A distinctly different, yet complementary, road to
traditional mindfulness. Where traditional approaches
focus primarily on 'doing and practicing,' (and we
incorporate some of those elements), I also encourage
an 'as-needed, as-inspired, as-inclined' approach,
allowing mindfulness to naturally weave into your day
without a rigid schedule, where I invite you to relax in the
direct experience of 'now,' (especially in later chapters),
revealing and resting in the light of open, gentle spacious
awareness that is always shining, the space before
thought arises, which I believe is as natural and integral
to our being as breathing. We understand that this is a
different approach than the MBSR community, teachers,
programs, and approaches who we hold in the highest
regard, and appreciate their excellent approach that is
perfect for many, we simply follow a different, and what
we believe to be a complementary, path.

• **Non-Bias (Embracing and Allowing vs. Non-
Judgment):** I invite an "embracing and allowing what
arises" as an effortless receptive observation, gently
navigating biases, thought patterns, emotional habits,
and reactive responses. This allows us to freely ride the
waves of perception and life experience rather than being
derailed or unduly influenced by them. While deeply
respecting the traditional mindfulness approaches and
community, and while there are many layers of shared
values, our approach embraces the non-active aspect of

the traditional "nonjudgement" tenet, which we refer to as a 'receptive without-bias' approach.

• **Revealing, Not Seeking (Inherent Wisdom):** The ideas of a relaxed, easy, and comfortable approach, gently settling into wisdom's natural embrace, naturally revealed, not actively pursued are also part of what I present in this book. Traditional approaches offer valuable tools and proven methods, and we acknowledge their many contributions, yet what I present is a slightly alternative approach where 'revealing' inherent wisdom is a foundational perspective.

• **Non-Action, No Agenda (Effortless Being):** In some exercises, I invite you to settle into experiences of natural perfection, releasing the internal knots and fierce grip of upset, allowing thoughts and sensations to arise and unfold with natural ease, without aim or agenda. And while I recognize the value of practice-oriented mindfulness programs, and understand that they have successfully served and supported many people withenriching experiences, I am presenting a path that emphasizes 'effortless being.'

• **Mindfulness vs. Mindlessness (Pre-Thinking Awareness):** As you'll see in the upcoming text, I explore and expand on this subtle idea. We can simply relax, rest, and settle into spacious open awareness—the "before the thinking mind intervenes" that underlies our our matrix of bias, preference, and agenda. I invite you to explore the spaciousness of awareness that exists before thought, allowing biases and agendas to naturally dissolve. I applaud and acknowledge the transformative power of concentration-heavy approaches, and while they serve many needs, we offer another option that explores the spaciousness of pre-thinking awareness.

• **Natural Perfection, Inherent Wholeness (Beyond Imperfection):** Occasionally, I weave in the idea of the inherent wholeness of our being, inviting you to relax and settle into boundless natural purity. And while I deeply appreciate the wide-spread adoption of medical and therapy-based mindfulness by the professional healthcare community, as well as their impressive contributions and advancements in this field of health and wellness, I see this approach as a complementary perspective focused on inherent wholeness.

• **Dzogchen and Vajrayana Inspired (Wisdom-Driven, Not Spiritual):** The presented approach is informed by these rich traditions, emphasizing the immediacy and inherent availability of clear unbiased awareness, but always clearly presented in a straightforward manner, using non-spiritual, non-dogmatic, simple language to present the concepts, the practical in-life contexts, and how to easily and seamlessly integrate it all into daily life at the level of your need or desire.

• **Life-Centric, Not Practice-Centric:** I have tried to elaborate on the idea that mindfulness is a life tool for everyday living. A tool for meeting all of life head-on, in all its glory, messiness, passion, upset, challenge, and joy—a whole-life approach. Mindfulness is our natural ticket to "embrace all of life" and not shy away, and show how it is mor ethan just a set of techniques to be practiced.

• **No-Meditation Required (Beyond Formal Practice):** I understand this is a bold statement. Let me say that there is nothing wrong with meditation, formal, guided, or casual, and even the more nuanced non-meditation approaches are a fantastic tool and I encourage anyone so inclined to jump in without any reservation!

> ◇ The option I present is not that one of "meditation" as a requirment, even though I do include some lovely visualization meditations. The goal is shift the burden of a "meditation requirement to something that is optiona, Even research has shown that "meditation" can significant barrier to mindfulness engagement for seniors, especially those without any meditation experience, Meditation can also act as a polarizing element to those considering exploring mindfulness, even leading to ideas of "exceptionalism" if "done well" or failure if not done "well enough," adding to the list of obstacles of adoption or continued engagement, especially for those in their later years.

◇ This is one of the main reasons. In my view, many people, perhaps including you, dear reader, may avoid mindfulness entirely or not continue with it, simply due to the "meditation requirement," time commitment, rigor, or the sentiment that "you won't get results without meditation," presented by other mindfulness schools, approaches, and clinical settings.

◇ **Our approach attempts to heal this rift,** bridging the gap for those who "can't" or "don't want to" meditate. **We say: Let's re-frame mindfulness into something inclusive, life-affirming, and accessible.** Meditate or don't, it doesn't matter from our perspective—instead, relax and release the knots of thoughts, emotions, and resistance, embrace the winds of change.

Settle into the flow of experience.

With mental and emotional notions relaxing,
ease and contentment are naturally revealed.

~ Inspired by traditional wisdom on a mindful approach.

Ultimately there is no "right" way, no required way, no "shoulds" or "musts" in our approach. You are free to adapt the techniques to suit your individual needs and preferences. We invite you to discover a path of mindfulness that is as unique and individual as you are. All we ask is that you consider allowing us to walk beside you as, together, we explore an all-of-life approach. We know it's not for everyone, but for those inclined, it is a delicious journey.

Why This Matters:

In essence, this approach is designed to be adaptable and accessible. I have intentionally set aside "should dos," "must dos," checklists, timers, certificates, and notions of striving. I present mindfulness as a simple, natural, effective, and even enjoyable life tool for anyone inclined to gently shift their inner dialogue, re-frame their experience of upheaval or discomfort, or savor life's richness in ways other approaches may overlook. This book was written and designed specifically with seniors in mind because I fully understand and appreciate the unique life challenges that may arise later in life, including the varied levels of uncertainty, discomfort, mobility issues, loss of independence, chronic pain, social isolation, anxiety, grief, and the desire to reclaim our mental and emotional resilience and stability. This book is just one of the Life Tools for Seniors I am creating to support those traveling their later years in meaningful and life-affirming ways.

Our Foundational Touchstones:

- "Just one breath" can be enough.

- Mindfulness is something that can be engaged by anyone, anytime.

- Mindfulness can be presented as a flexible, adaptable, and personalized life tool that is relevant and simple.

Designed specifically for seniors and these foundational touchstones in mind, creating an easy, flexible, adaptable, practical, and relevant approach to mindfulness.

Table 1: Subjective Comparison of Mindfulness, Related Practices & Approaches:

Formal & Rigqrous			Monastic and/or Zen
			Mindfulness Lifestyle
Medium Diffculty	Tai Chi/Qigong Asanas/Yoga	Secular: MBSR	Breathwork Vipassana
Simple Informal On-Demand	Our Approach	Secular: Hypnosis	Metta/Kindness Meditations
	Relaxing Enjoyable	Clinical Therapeutic	Goal Oriented

Table 2: The Mindfulness Spectrum—From Micro-Moments to Monastic Practice

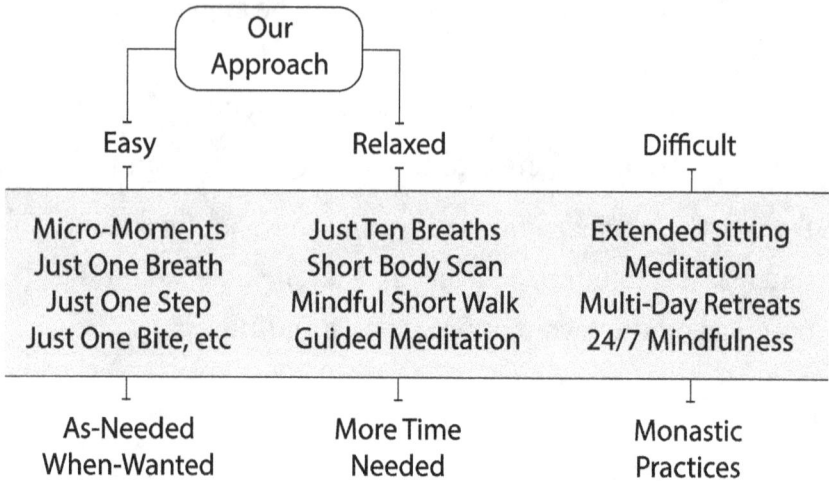

Our Approach		
Easy	Relaxed	Difficult
Micro-Moments Just One Breath Just One Step Just One Bite, etc	Just Ten Breaths Short Body Scan Mindful Short Walk Guided Meditation	Extended Sitting Meditation Multi-Day Retreats 24/7 Mindfulness
As-Needed When-Wanted	More Time Needed	Monastic Practices

Table 3: The Mindfulness Spectrum—Everyday Activities with Different Approaches

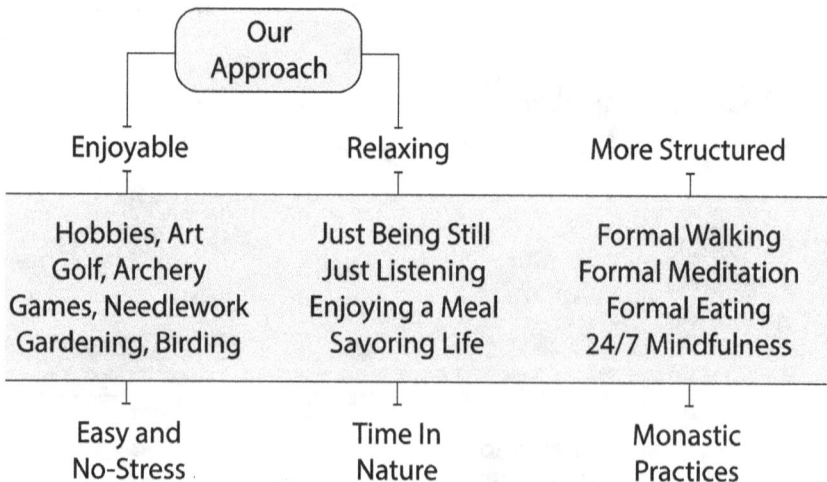

Our Approach		
Enjoyable	Relaxing	More Structured
Hobbies, Art Golf, Archery Games, Needlework Gardening, Birding	Just Being Still Just Listening Enjoying a Meal Savoring Life	Formal Walking Formal Meditation Formal Eating 24/7 Mindfulness
Easy and No-Stress	Time In Nature	Monastic Practices

Table 4: The Mindfulness Potential—Meeting Life's Challenges

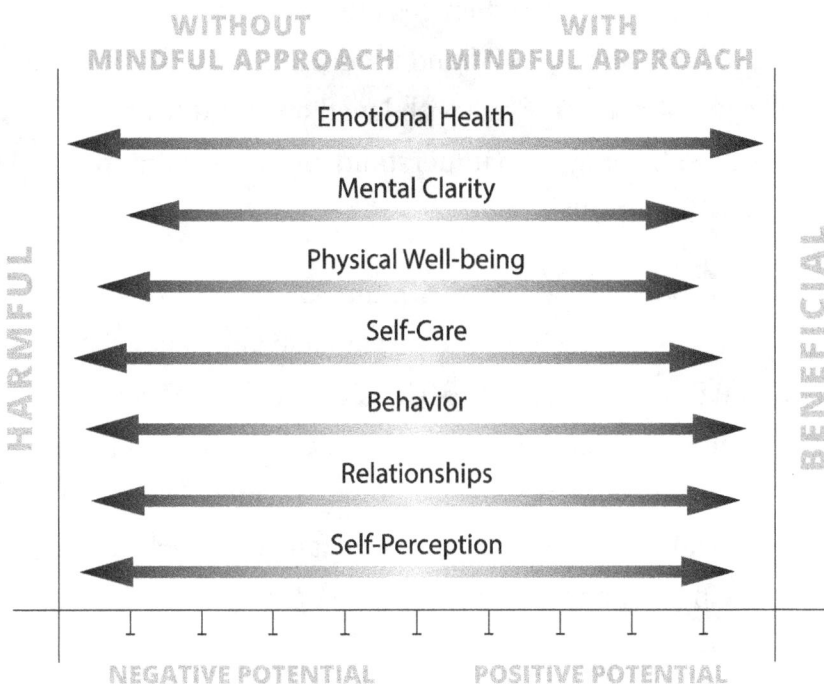

WITHOUT MINDFUL APPROACH   WITH MINDFUL APPROACH

HARMFUL

Emotional Health

Mental Clarity

Physical Well-being

Self-Care

Behavior

Relationships

Self-Perception

BENEFICIAL

NEGATIVE POTENTIAL   POSITIVE POTENTIAL

II. Who's This Book For?

So, who's this book for? Well, it's primarily written for folks aged 55 and beyond—that sweet spot in life where things start to shift and change for us. It's a time when we're looking for new ways to keep our bodies, minds, and spirits in good shape and a stage of life that can bring all sorts of new challenges and dramatic shifts to how we live and relate to the world. But it's also a time with great potential for incredible personal growth and self-discovery, as well as a deepening appreciation for all the experiences life has given.

Enter this mindfulness companion... a helpful ally on this journey of life, a trustworthy partner that can not only help us navigate life's challenges but also deepen our joy. Mindfulness, when viewed and used as a Life Tool, can help us deepen our connections with loved ones and friends, while also allowing us to understand and connect more deeply with ourselves.

While the book was written with the 55+ age group in mind, the practices and techniques are valuable and beneficial for individuals of any age or experiencing any life challenge. This includes, as my wife has pointed out, women in the 45+ age range who may be navigating hormonal shifts and the associated emotional and body changes, as well as new care-giving responsibilities with aging parents, and I believe many more as well.

Generally speaking, here are some benefits that mindfulness can offer, especially for us seniors:

• **Stress Reduction:** Mindfulness can help us meet and manage our age-related stress and anxiety, allowing for a calmer approach to life—soothing and comforting, like a gentle cool breeze on a hot summer day.

• **Improved Sleep:** Mindfulness techniques, supported by both my own experience and scientific research, can improve sleep quality and lead to more restful nights— and who doesn't want to wake up feeling refreshed and ready to embrace the day?

- **Enhanced Cognitive Function:** Emerging research suggests that mindfulness can support cognitive health, helping us keep our minds sharp and engaged—like a well-oiled machine.

- **Emotional Well-being:** Mindfulness offers strategies and tools to build a more resilient emotional landscape, reducing reactivity and anger, and promoting calmer, more insightful responses. It nurtures our own sense of peace and contentment—a tool for more gracefully navigating life's inevitable twists and turns.

- **Connection and Joy:** One of the less-often-mentioned benefits of mindfulness is its ability to deepen our connections with others and ourselves, enriching our lives and allowing us to truly savor and appreciate all that life offers, both in the everyday moments and the special events.

Why This Book?

A Personal Journey and a Shared Experience

As a senior myself, I've come to realize that many of the emotional and physical challenges I've faced—such as varying degrees of anxiety, fear, anger, frustration, as well as physical traumas with extended periods of recovery and rehabilitation—are likely shared by others in this stage of life. This book stems from decades of personal experience navigating these very issues, and finding solutions for a more meaningful and happier life. I believe the tools and approaches I've learned can be of great benefit to fellow seniors.

I understand that not everyone will be drawn to mindfulness, but for those who are, I believe it offers a powerful way to enhance mental, emotional, and physical well-being. Moreover, these tools, exercises, and techniques have the potential to positively transform our relationships—with our partners, families, friends, colleagues, and even casual acquaintances.

From Challenge to Transformation

My inspiration for writing this book comes from my own experiences with difficulty, loss, frustration, and anger. Like many others, I've been overwhelmed by my own emotional responses at times. However, I've also experienced breakthroughs and transformations—not grand, world-altering changes, but simple yet profound shifts in how I react to life. I've learned to manage anger more effectively, cultivate greater patience, and become more open to life's inevitable ups and downs.

These personal challenges are often amplified by the uncertainties of the world around us. While this book isn't a magic solution to remove all our cares, it does offer ways to work with the "flames" of our charged emotional states and reactions. It gives us tools to address and even heal the heated response or anger that arises when we feel thrown off balance by a situation, and also reset and heal the habitual reactions that we so often later regret. My hope is that these tools will be helpful, enjoyable, and beneficial for anyone who chooses to explore them.

The Author's Personal Mindfulness Journey

Like many of us, I've faced my share of life's curve-balls. One experience, in particular, dramatically reshaped my life and ultimately led me to an extended exploration of mindfulness. At the age of 30, I was involved in a serious motor vehicle accident—a head-on collision with a drunk driver. The aftermath was a whirlwind of legal, physical, and emotional challenges resulting from injuries I sustained including numerous fractures, lacerations, internal injuries, and a significant head injury with cognitive deficits, and the resulting surgeries and rehabilitation efforts.

The impact of this event rippled through every aspect of my life. I faced 18 months of physical therapy just to regain the use of my leg and relearn how to walk. I had to adapt to diminished lung capacity and, for over a year, I had to navigate the world with walkers, canes and other assistive devices. I also struggled with the emotional fallout—PTSD, anger, frustration, and a diminished sense of self-worth. In short, the "Blair" I knew before the crash was forced to confront and rebuild a "new Blair."

This experience, though deeply challenging, became a catalyst for personal growth. It forced me to confront my limitations, to surrender to circumstances beyond my control, and to seek out new ways of coping and healing. It was during this time that I renewed and expanded my efforts with mindfulness as a way to help me manage my new life situation, as much out of necessity as it was an intentional choice. Mindfulness became a way to re-embody and reinvent myself, to find peace amidst the chaos, and beauty amongst the ashes, and to navigate the labyrinth of physical, mental, and emotional pain.

My story, while unique to me, is not about exceptionalism. It's about the common human experience of facing adversity and finding ways to move forward. It's about recognizing that even in the face of significant challenges, it's possible to find peace, resilience, and even joy. Mindfulness became one of the tools that helped me rebuild my life, and it continues to be a source of strength and well-being to this day. My hope is that by sharing this part of my journey, I can offer hope, encouragement, and connection to others, especially seniors who may be facing their own unique set of challenges and adversity. Mindfulness, I've discovered, can be a valuable part of the healing and aging process—a tasty tool to enjoy the pie we call life.

IV. How to Use This Book

This book is designed to be both a guided journey through the core principles of mindfulness and a practical resource you can turn to whenever you need it. It's structured to help you progressively deepen your understanding of mindfulness—moving from no prior experience to a functional grasp of key concepts—but feel free to use it in whatever way best serves you.

Think of it as your personal mindfulness toolkit. You can read it cover to cover, dive into specific chapters as needed, or simply grab the book for a quick exercise when life throws a curve-ball. Whether you're just looking for basic breath exercises, need some strategies to navigate emotional upheaval, tools for working with physical discomfort, or support in navigating life changes or personal loss, this book is here to help. Please feel free to read the material and use the exercises as needed and at your own pace because adapting and flexing the content to your needs and situation is key.

Trying the Techniques:

This book isn't just about reading; it's about doing and engaging the process. While we encourage you to try the mindfulness exercises suggested throughout the book, we also suggest starting small, perhaps with just a few minutes of mindful breathing each day (even one mindful breath is a great start!), and gradually increasing the duration of your engagement as you become more familiar and comfortable with the ideas and techniques. Remember, there's no right or wrong way to engage with mindfulness. The most important thing is to approach each exercise with an open mind and a gentle, accepting attitude (and remember to be kind to yourself—it really is a journey, and not a performance or something with a test to evaluate your prowess).

Navigation and Support:

For easy book navigation, I have included a detailed table of contents at the beginning of each chapter, in addition to the comprehensive table of contents at the front of the book. Exercises are grouped at the end of longer chapters so you can quickly find them without searching through the text. You'll also find detailed background information and explanations on a range of topics, including mindfulness, health challenges, pain and discomfort, and emotional well-being. Our goal is to provide you with the information and support you need on your journey.

No-Glossary Approach:

Key concepts in mindfulness are best understood through their detailed exploration within the book's chapters. Please use the comprehensive index to locate discussions of key terms in their full context.

Keeping a Mindfulness Journal (or Using Our Mindfulness Tracker):

To enhance your mindfulness journey, one tool we have enjoyed using from time to time is a mindfulness journal. This can be a simple notebook where you jot down your experiences, insights, and reflections after each effort or exercise, or at the end of your day. In this journal, you might note how you felt before, during, and after the exercise, any thoughts or emotions that arose, and any insights you gained about the effects you felt during the course of the day.

For those who prefer a more structured approach, we've also created a 30-Day Mindfulness Tracker (available late June or early July, 2025, as a separate book or a downloadable resource). This tracker provides prompts and exercises to guide your daily mindfulness explorations to help you track your experiences and shifts over time. Using a journal or tracker can provide valuable insights into your own unique mindfulness journey and help you deepen your understanding and integration of these techniques.

Ultimately, this book is for you, dear reader. Use it in whatever way best supports you on your journey of challenge, growth, and exploration of mindfulness.

May You Find Your Mindfulness Adventure To Be Relevant, Helpful & Enjoyable!

V. What You'll Find in This Book:

This book is structured to provide a comprehensive and practical guide to mindfulness for seniors. What follows is a brief overview of what you'll find in each book section:

Part 1: Foundations of Practical Mindfulness (Chapters 1-2): These introductory chapters lay the groundwork for your mindfulness explorations, exploring essential concepts such as:

- The Power of the Here and Now
- Understanding the Mind
- Understanding the Body-Mind Connection
- And more...

Part 2: Tools and Techniques (Chapters 3-6): This section offers step-by-step instructions for a variety of practical mindfulness techniques, including:

- Mindful Breathing
- Body Scan Meditation
- Mindful Walking
- Mindful Eating
- Visualizations
- And more...

Part 3: Mindfulness for Specific Life Stages and Challenges (Chapters 7-10): These chapters explore how mindfulness can be applied to specific challenges faced by seniors, such as:

- Managing pain and health concerns
- Coping with grief, loss, and life transitions
- Reducing anxiety and stress
- Mindfulness in relationships and senior safety
- Embracing gratitude and joy
- And more...

Other Support and Resources:

I believe that support is essential for cultivating a sustainable and meaningful mindfulness engagement. To that end, I have created several resources (most are free and other very low cost) to help you along your journey:

As of this books publishing date, available resources include:

- A mindfulness journal/tracker
- Companion book "100 Mindful Moments for Seniors"
- Senior-specific mindfulness articles (by the author)
- Links to senior-specific mindfulness resources/research
- "Inspired by Joy" bi-weekly newsletter
- Educational and Inspiring content and videos
- Private individual and small group coaching

Planned future resources:

- Private Online group(s)
- Online and Pre-recorded Classes
- Custom and Prerecorded Classes
- Mindfulness support tools
- Other books/booklets on mindfulness for Seniors
- Mindfulness App designed for Seniors

Use Cases and Examples:

To give you a better idea of how you can integrate mindfulness into your daily life, here are a few examples:

- **Morning Routine:** Start your day with a short mindful breathing exercise (Chapter 4) to set a calm and focused tone for the day (it's a great way to set the tone of your day).

- **Managing Pain:** If you're experiencing chronic or episodic pain, refer to the chapter on mindfulness for pain management (Chapter 8) for specific techniques to help you cope with discomfort (remember, mindfulness isn't about eliminating pain, though for many, it can help to lessen it, it is more about changing your relationship to it... and of course, if additional pain support is needed, we always encourage you to work with your health practitioners for supplemental pain support if needed).

• **Dealing with Loneliness:** When feeling lonely or disconnected, explore the exercises in the chapter on mindfulness for connection and relationships (Chapter 10) to cultivate a sense of belonging, connection, and calmness in the face of any isolation you are experiencing (don't discount the tried-and-true "reaching out to others" and asking to meet or talk... not only can companionship help with feelings of isolation, it is also a rich ground for engaging mindfulness in a way that supports your growth and enrichment).

• **Before Bedtime:** Perform a body scan mindful meditation (Chapter 5) before bed to relax your body and mind and promote restful sleep (a good night's sleep can make all the difference and this can really help, either when going to sleep or when trying to get back to sleep).

• **During a Difficult Moment:** If you find yourself feeling overwhelmed or agitated during the day, take a few mindful breaths (Chapter 4) to anchor yourself in the present moment and regain a sense of calm (in time, this technique can become our best tool, a good friend, and a personal reset button).

• **In a waiting room:** While waiting for an appointment, try Mindful Observation (Chapter 7) to become in tune and aware of the present moment (waiting rooms can become a great opportunity for mindfulness explorations).

A Note on Adaptation:

Remember, the previous list are just suggestions. Feel free to adapt the techniques and approaches to suit your individual needs, abilities, and preferences.

If a particular exercise doesn't feel right for you, that's perfectly okay (mindfulness is about flexibility, not rigidity).

The goal is to find what works best for you and to create a meaningful and rewarding mindfulness approach that supports your well-being and your path forward.

Intro Section 2

"Mindfulness is like water—
it flows everywhere and can be
enjoyed anywhere by anyone,
regardless of their physical condition."

From "Mindfulness for Seniors"

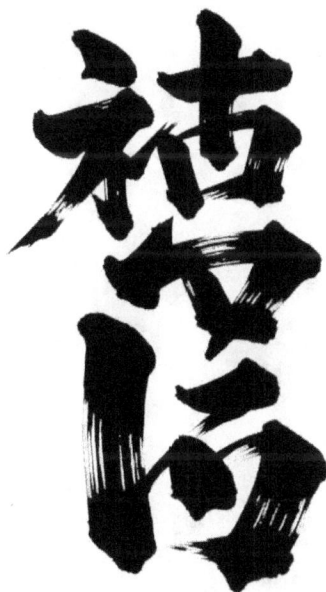

Core Concepts

TABLE OF CONTENTS for

INTRODUCTION PART TWO: CORE CONCEPTS

Introduction Part Two:
Core Concepts

"If you want to conquer the anxiety of life,
live in the moment, live in the breath."

- Amit Ray Ph.D.
(Author, speaker, teacher)

I. Welcome

Hello, and welcome. If you're holding this book in your hands (or a digital version), it's likely that you, like me, are navigating the unique landscape of our senior years. This stage of life, while filled with potential for wisdom, joy, and deeper connection, also brings its own set of transitions and adjustments—physical changes, lifestyle shifts, and accompanying emotional currents. Perhaps you've noticed that your body doesn't quite move with the same ease it once did, or maybe you're facing the loss of loved ones or adapting to a new life chapter. These experiences are a natural part of aging, and they can sometimes contribute to feelings of unease, apprehension, or a sense of estrangement.

In today's fast-paced world, it's easy to feel overwhelmed, agitated, and detached from ourselves, our friends, our family, our social circles, and disengaged from the present moment. This overwhelm and agitation, coupled with long-held habits of thought and emotional patterns—sometimes reinforced by external pressures—can often create what feels like unseen shackles that constrain our experience of the present. These constraints can manifest as worry, unease, physical discomfort, or a general sense of isolation from ourselves and the world around us. This book offers a path to recognizing and gently loosening these constraints, allowing you to experience life with greater awareness, freedom, and joy.

That path is mindfulness. And, mindfulness, as we'll explore in these pages, isn't about escaping life's difficulties; it's about meeting them with greater awareness, intention, and openness. It's a practical approach that can help us cultivate a calmer, more focused mind, allowing us to savor the present moment and find greater contentment, even amidst life's uncertainties.

This book isn't a quick fix or a magic wand. It's a practical toolkit—a collection of simple yet powerful exercises and techniques that you can adapt, reshape, and tweak to suit your own unique needs and preferences. It's an invitation to embark on a journey of self-discovery, a journey that can lead to greater peace, resilience, and a deeper appreciation for the life you've lived and the life you continue to live.

II. Why Mindfulness for Seniors?

As we journey through life, we accumulate a rich tapestry of experiences—joys, sorrows, triumphs, and setbacks—that shape the personality we present to ourselves and the world. These experiences, both big and small, can create deeply ingrained patterns of thinking, feeling, and reacting. While some of these habits serve us well, others can become a source of stress, anxiety, emotional outbursts, discontent, blaming, regrets, and a sense of disconnection from who we truly are and the world around us. This is especially true as we navigate the unique terrain of our senior years, a time of both wonderful opportunities and significant transitions. Mindfulness offers a gentle and effective way to navigate these challenges with greater awareness, intention, and self-compassion, allowing us to choose a new path beyond automatic reactions.

Beyond Automatic Reactions: Choosing a New Path

We don't have to be stuck in our automatic reactive responses. We have a choice, even in seemingly small moments, when someone cuts us off in traffic, takes our parking spot, is abrupt or rude to us, or makes a mistake with our order. These choices, both large and small, either reinforce old, unhelpful patterns or pave a path toward the more peaceful and fulfilling life we envision. This applies equally to major life events—a difficult diagnosis, the loss of a loved one, or the consequences of our mistakes—and to the daily mini-irritations that inevitably arise. This book offers a practical toolkit for making more conscious and intentional decisions—decisions that counter habitual emotional responses like anger, anxiety, or agitation, decisions that help us reset our reactive habits and broaden our perspectives. Many of these automatic responses stem from past traumas, frustrations, or repeated challenges that have shaped our personalities, for better or worse. These ingrained patterns can operate on autopilot, often below our level of awareness, creating challenging experiences for ourselves and others. But there's a better way forward, a way to cultivate greater ease and well-being, both for ourselves and for the quality of our relationships.

Addressing the Unique Challenges and Opportunities of Aging

Aging presents a unique blend of challenges and opportunities. As I've moved into my seventh decade, these have become increasingly clear. Many of us experience physical changes—body systems that don't function as they once did, potential declines in mental acuity, memory loss, sleep, and eating difficulties, and many small and larger challenges in every aspect of daily life. These physical changes can often be compounded by cultural challenges, such as feeling less valued or respected by family members or society or facing skill deficits related to vision, balance, or mobility. Past and current illnesses, traumas, or surgeries can further complicate our path. This book acknowledges these realities with empathy and understanding and offers practical support for navigating this important stage of life. It encourages us to savor the life we have, cultivate gratitude for the present moment, and meet challenges with a calm and focused mind. It's about gently allowing our best selves to emerge, all while fully embracing life's uncertainties and the realities that accompany those circumstances, including the finite nature of life itself. By cultivating a clearer, brighter, and less reactive mind, we can move through life in ways that are more spontaneous, more relaxed, increasingly joyful, and more beneficial both to ourselves and to those we cherish.

III. Mindfulness: A Practical, Flexible & Adaptable Life Tool

Understanding Mindfulness: More Than Meets the Eye

Mindfulness, as a concept, encompasses a wide variety of approaches and techniques. Even in my own early efforts to understand it, I found the idea quite confusing. Questions like "Is mindfulness the same as meditation?" (Spoiler alert: no, they are not the same, though they do overlap) can be intimidating for those considering mindfulness. Adding to the confusion, many people, whether intentionally or not, pigeonhole mindfulness into rigid definitions, depending on their perspectives, preferences, experiences, or even fears.

A Spectrum of Possibilities: Finding What Works for You

In my experience, mindfulness is best understood as a spectrum of techniques, approaches, structures, and styles— everything from simple, fleeting, easy-to-try momentary acts to more involved and structured formal practices, and everything in between. This adaptability and flexibility is what makes mindfulness a fantastic option for anyone and particularly well-suited to seniors. Whether you're dealing with physical challenges or limitations, struggling with overwhelming emotions, facing mental acuity challenges, or simply wanting to savor life's moments, mindfulness can offer support. Mindfulness can also provide valuable tools for managing common negative thought patterns, including negative self-talk, low self-esteem, a consistently negative outlook, or a tendency to be overly critical. All of these are perfect starting points for experiencing mindfulness.

Mindfulness Can Be Joyful and Light

Another important aspect is that mindfulness doesn't have to be difficult or even serious. To the surprise of many, it can be playful, uplifting, and joyful, even rejuvenating and energizing, and more. From my perspective, this notion of "serious practice" seems based on monastic traditions. And while these cloistered formal practices are perfect for some, they are not a perfect fit for everyone, especially seniors! So, if "serious" is not your thing, go ahead and lighten up and have a laugh. If you want to simply smile and enjoy your day or outing, perfect! This is what I call the hidden superpower of mindfulness: no matter what you are doing, no matter what stage of life you are in, mindfulness can be a diamond in your pocket—something of great value that you can always carry with you.

IV. What is Mindfulness?

The Confusing and Seemingly Contradictory Mindfulness Definitions

Let's be honest, trying to figure out what mindfulness really is can be a real head-scratcher. There's so much conflicting information out there. Depending on who you talk to—or which book you read—mindfulness can be presented in wildly different ways. This adds to the confusion, making it seem like there's a "right" way and a "wrong" way to not only work with mindfulness but also to understand its core principles. And to make things even more confusing, some people use "mindfulness" and "meditation" interchangeably as if they're the same thing, while others see them as distinct techniques.

An Alternative Way to Think About Mindfulness (and Meditation)

I've found it helpful to think of mindfulness and meditation as having two distinct approaches: one involving intentional effort and the other a more effortless approach. We can call these "With Effort" and "Without Effort." The "With Effort" approach refers to focused techniques with mindfulness and meditation, where we intentionally direct our attention. The "Without Effort" approach, simply put, is the experience of our basic awareness before conscious thought arises. This is not the same as being inattentive, in a trance, or unaware; rather, it's a state of relaxed, spacious awareness.

Beyond Doing to Being

Another way of engaging and experiencing "Being" or pure awareness, is to simply "relax." When I say "relax," I'm referring to both our body and our mind—our thoughts, opinions, judgments, preferences, and so on. In Chapters 4 through 7, we will explore some simple techniques that will help with this transition from "doing" to "being."

Ultimately, remember that there is no single "right" way to engage with mindfulness. Whether you approach it with focused effort or gentle ease, whatever your current capacity or experience, the path is yours alone. Trust that any progress or insights will naturally unfold, just like the morning mists under the face of the rising sun. Mindfulness offers the potential to cultivate greater personal contentment, ease, and even joy in our daily lives, allowing us not only to experience the richness of the present moment but also to navigate all of life's situations— the happy times and the not-so-happy times—with greater confidence and grace.

V. Exploring Aspects of Mindfulness

Mindfulness (with Effort)

A Gentle Nudge of Awareness

This aspect of mindfulness serves as a foundational technique, a central hub from which other approaches branch out. It's based on intention and choice, offering tools for both navigating challenging circumstances and cultivating deeper experiences of gratitude, happiness, and joy. While we use the word "effort," it's more of a gentle nudge of awareness than an arduous undertaking. This gentle approach makes it particularly well-suited for seniors, as even minimal effort can create space to reset reactivity to difficult emotions and deepen positive feelings.

Practical Examples for Daily Life:

The approaches I present begin with simple, accessible activities like "one breath," "one bite," or "one step," which can be done anywhere. The biggest challenge is simply remembering to try it a few times throughout the day. A helpful extension is what I call the "Rule of 3's"—taking three breaths, three bites, or three steps mindfully. This slight increase can significantly enhance awareness. However, "easy does it" is key. These exercises should never feel burdensome or irritating; think "savor," as a way to enjoy the process.

While extended sessions of breath-watching, mindful walks, or slow, methodical eating can be beneficial, especially for those drawn to a deeper dive, it's essential to approach them with gentleness and awareness of any resistance that may arise (mental, emotional, or physical). Slow and steady progress is the best approach. Remember to observe any arising inner critic as just another thought to notice and then let recede, like a wave returning to the sea.

Mindfulness in the Face of Challenges:

When using mindfulness "with effort" to work with challenging emotions, the focus shifts from "savoring" to "standing strong," "confidently facing," or simply "being brave enough to sit in the heat of the moment and just breathe." The idea is to allow the emotions, racing thoughts, and bodily sensations to wash over you like a breaking wave that eventually recedes, doing your best to simply notice your reactions and just breathe until calmness or clarity can be had. Importantly, remember that sometimes the most mindful action is to create distance from a challenging situation—by leaving the room, ending a conversation, or stepping away to regain composure.

The Potential of Mindfulness (with Effort) for Seniors:

For seniors, simplicity and gentleness are paramount— gentleness in body, speech, and mind. When engaged with earnest intention (a gentle, nudging earnestness), these techniques pose no threat to one's established personality or sense of self. Instead, they enrich the person, fostering a gentler, kinder, and more integrated approach to life. In this context, mindfulness is like a marinade, deepening the flavors and enriching the quality of life, even—and perhaps especially—in the face of challenges. Seniors may experience a sense of peace, calmness, greater equanimity, gratitude, joy, and contentment—both in pleasurable experiences and during less savory times. These positive effects may sometimes be felt immediately, but often they emerge after the intensity of a difficult moment or situation has passed.

Challenging Concepts Ahead:

Go slow with next section. It"s a bit nuanced. I have done my best to make this information clear and simply a point of reference. This is not something to strive for... just a note that this may be something you experience when engaging or relaxing into mindfulness.

Mindfulness (Without Effort)

Relaxing into Spacious Awareness

Here I begin to explore a side of mindfulness that is not often addressed. It's about the side of mindfulness where the present moment awareness is so complete and immersive that there is no longer a "doer" (or sense of self) engaging with a mindful activity. Our word for this state is 'Mindlessness' – a natural state, perhaps akin to being 'without self-consciousness,' where awareness is spacious and pre-thought. The way I use the term here, is not to be confused with a state of inattentiveness or entering a trance-like state. Inattentiveness implies mental distraction, while "trance" has various interpretations, some of which are unrelated to mindfulness.

Rather, Mindlessness is natural state... something that is revealed rather than achieved... it is more about relaxing into an expanded, spacious, pre-thought awareness of the present moment, allowing the sensory worlds (the perception of internal and external perceptions) to simply arise.

A key characteristic of this state is "aimlessness"—not in the sense of lacking purpose in life, but rather in the sense of "no effort, no agenda, no-bias" in the present moment.

It can be occur one of two ways:

1. As a natural transition/progression/release from mindful techniques (with effort)

2. Or as spontaneously arising awareness of the panoramic totality of experience. (without effort)

Another way to think about Mindlessness:

Think of mindlessness like the sun that is always shining behind the clouds – And just like how the sun is always shining, so too, our natural state of pure awareness is always present, but it's often obscured by the 'clouds' of our thoughts, worries, and habitual patterns.

While the experience of mindlessness can arise at any time, just like when the 'clouds' spontaneously part and reveal the sun, there really isn't a way to force them to part. It's more about a gradual 'relaxing of the mind,' a gentle loosening of our firm grasp on the world as we perceive it. And in this example, the tighter our grasp, the more 'stuck' the clouds become.

This 'letting go' is a process, and it can be challenging due to our ingrained mental habits, constant conceptualizing, and our emotional needs or feelings.

However, familiarization with mindfulness techniques, cultivating deep relaxation, and engaging in activities with such mindful focus that we momentarily forget about the self – these can all be seen as ways that may create the conditions for the 'clouds of that block the sun' to part, revealing glimpses of a genuine relaxed and natural state of awareness.

It's natural and nothing to fear—simply a temporary perceptual shift. I like to think of it as our foundational awareness peeking through... and place of childlike wonder and awe... that place that is just enjoying before our thoughts arise.

Good, Better, Best?

It's important to understand that neither of these states are "better" or "righter" than others; they are simply different facets of experience. The beauty of simple mindful techniques (with effort) is that it often leads to this effortless, spacious awareness. There's no need to strive for a "superior state" or achieve a specific level. The basic act of mindfulness, when fully engaged, can naturally transition into this non-effort flow state of relaxed awareness.

Just Be Here Now:

The key is to simply relax into what unfolds in your perceptions. There's no need to worry about reaching some "better place"; just be here now! As Thich Nhat Hanh says, "This is the Pure Land."

That said, the "with-effort techniques" can act like a "magic trick," allow us to relax our grip on our "story" and the narratives of "me and mine," softening the knots of our emotional upsets and habitual thinking.

VI. Understanding Meditation and Mindfulness

Meditation / Mindfulness: Key Differences

Let's explore the concept of meditation and how it differs from mindfulness, at least from our perspective and how we approach this in this book. Traditional meditation, whether from Eastern or Western spiritual traditions, is generally a structured, intentional practice, often performed in a seated or kneeling position. Each session has a beginning (often with "preliminaries"), a progression, and an end, typically within a timed session or framework. Most meditations engage the conscious mind and mental focus and may include specific rules, cultural formalities, visualizations, or recitations. In contrast, mindfulness is much more simple and direct, with a focus, with or without effort, on the present moment as it unfolds. It can be as simple as focusing on one relaxed breath. Meditation tends to be goal-oriented (achieving a specific state or outcome), while mindfulness embraces and dances with the present moment. The phrase "no place to go, nothing to do, and no time other than the present" offers a taste of the immediacy of mindfulness.

Meditation / Mindfulness: Adaptability for Seniors

While this book focuses on mindfulness, formal meditation postures can be adapted as needed to our exercises if you are familiar with them. However, a key aspect of mindfulness is its inherent flexibility. It removes the constraints of specific postures and positions, emphasizing what is comfortable for you. While meditation often emphasizes specific postures (like full or half lotus for instance or particular breathing practices), mindfulness can be engaged while in any posture or during any activity, whether you prefer sitting on a chair, standing, or evenmoving or performing tasks. I believe, especially when it comes to my fellow seniors, simply using everyday postures like sitting, kneeling, walking, leaning, or resting are best. Even a simple breath or two while engaged in some daily activity, noticing the feel of a mug in your hand, or appreciating the view from your front steps can be a gateway to wonderful world. While structured formalities are often associated with traditional meditation, they are not required for developing mindfulness and can be set aside to lighten the load of expectations. Crooked posture? Don't worry about it! Got a limp? Me too! Mindfulness is like water—it flows everywhere and can be enjoyed anywhere by anyone, regardless of their physical condition.

Meditation / Mindfulness: The "Doing" Approach

The "doing approach" encompasses both what I am calling "Active Meditation" and "Active Mindfulness". This is where someone is engaged by choice and is acting with intention, usually following specific procedures and instructions. My focus though is to make the exercises accessible and easy to use.

Functionally, mindfulness is just a focused present-moment awareness, following a more open approach than the formal meditation approaches. A relaxed present-moment awareness with no time extension, no goal, no level to achieve—nothing to do other than "be aware" and fully present (as much as our capacities allow).

While effort-based active meditation, even if only for a few minutes, involves distinct steps: starting, doing, and stopping. Mindfulness, on the other hand, is more of a continuous flow, like a stream that is constantly flowing and changing as it passes, yet forever ungraspable.

Meditation / Mindfulness: The Overlap

Meditation, when performed properly, is very mindful. Conversely, mindfulness naturally embodies a meditative quality. Mindfulness is like skipping the meditation preliminaries and jumping right into the heart of the meditation experience but without the rules, steps, visualizations, or prayers of formal meditation. Mindfulness is direct; it cuts to the heart of the matter... right now! It's like embarking on an ocean cruise but leaving all your mental and emotional luggage on the dock, sailing away into the present moment.

Anyone who stops learning is old, whether at twenty or eighty. Anyone who keeps learning stays young."

~ Henry Ford

VII. Doing & Being: A Spectrum of Experience

Mindfulness and Meditation: The "Doing"

Mindfulness (with effort) and Meditation (Structured Practice) both involve active engagement—a "doing." They are techniques we intentionally engage in, involving choice, intention, and specific actions. These approaches can be valuable tools for seniors, providing a way to interrupt negative self-talk, gain new perspectives, and even promote positive changes in the brain and body.

Effortless Awareness:: The "Being"

This shift from active engagement to a state of simply "being," resting in spaciousness beyond internal chatter, as mentioned, can either arise spontaneously, or as a natural result of consistent mindful or meditative techniques. **It's important to understand that these experiences are not something you can force or achieve through effort; rather, they are simply a revealing that unfolds when the grip of the self loosens.** It's like the unwinding of a spool of thread; when all the threads of self are no longer in play, effortless awareness is revealed.

The Value of Both Doing and Being

Both "doing" and "being" have value. For us seniors, the "doing" of mindfulness provides practical tools for navigating daily life, managing challenges, and cultivating well-being. The potential for "being"—resting in spaciousness—offers a deeper dimension of experience, a sense of peace and connection that transcends the limitations of the self.

However, it's crucial not to turn "being" into another goal to strive for. The quiet nudge of our focus should remain on the "gentle doing" of mindfulness. Sooner or later, as our mental and emotional grasp relaxes and releases, "being" may be naturally revealed.

It is not about actively 'creating conditions' to achieve a state of 'being.' Rather, it's about consistently, at whatever level youb are comfortable, to engage a mindful approach – the 'gentle doing' gradually loosens the grip of our habitual thought patterns and allows our natural relaxed awareness of 'being' to be revealed. Think of it like learning a musical instrument. You don't sit down with the goal of instantly becoming a virtuoso. Instead, you focus on the 'doing' – the consistent practice of scales, chords, and exercises. Over time, as your skill develops, moments of effortless musicality – the 'being' – naturally arise.

The "No-Self" Experience: A Sense of Interconnection

In moments of fully relaxed non-grasping awareness, the usual sense of a separate, individual "self" can soften, revealing a sense of interconnectedness with all things.

This isn't about denying your existence or becoming apathetic. It's more like realizing that you are part of something larger, like a wave in the ocean—distinct yet also connected to the vastness of the sea. This experience can bring a profound calm, ease, acceptance, and even joy.

Exploring Interconnectedness

The "no-self" experience, sometimes called "selflessness," "egolessness" or an "boundless sense of being," "Union with the Divine," and more, is a concept found in many spiritual traditions.

It's not about losing your identity; it's about recognizing that your sense of self is more fluid and interconnected than we often realize.

Think of a tree... It's a distinct individual tree, yet it's also part of the forest ecosystem, sharing resources and contributing to the whole. The "no-self" experience is similar—recognizing our individual existence while also understanding our deep connection to everything around us.

Experiencing Interconnectedness

This sense of interconnectedness isn't something you can force. It's a potential that can arise naturally when we release our grip on a fixed and solid sense of self.

It can happen during formal practices like mindfulness or meditation, or it can occur spontaneously in the activities of everyday life—during a moment of deep connection with a loved one, while gazing at a beautiful sunset, or simply while resting quietly.

For seniors, this experience can be particularly meaningful. As life transitions bring changes and losses, this sense of interconnectedness can offer a sense of perspective and acceptance, reminding us of the deeper unity of all things and providing a sense of peace that transcends the challenges of aging. It is a natural aspect of being, available to all, regardless of background or prior experience with mindfulness or meditation.

With these foundational core concepts in mind, we will be able to explore the practical applications of mindfulness in the main book chapters.

"Mindfulness is simply resting in what is already present—nothing to add or subtract."
~ Author

Intro Section 3

"One of the biggest obstacles
to mindfulness is our strong
attachment to our thoughts..."

From "Mindfulness for Seniors"

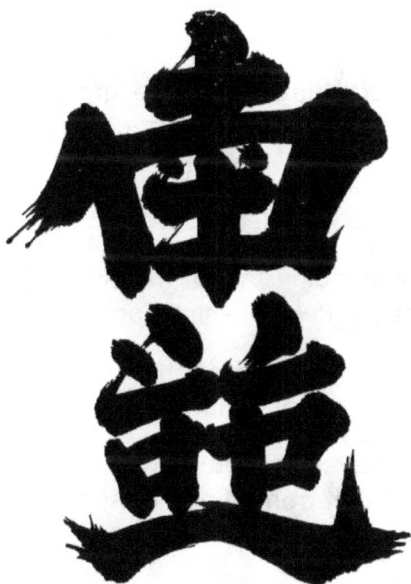

Obstacles & Misconceptions

TABLE OF CONTENTS for

INTRODUCTION PART THREE: COMMON MINDFULNESS
OBSTACLES, MISCONCEPTIONS, & MINDFULNESS HISTORY

Introduction Part Three:
Obstacles & Misconceptions

(& History)

"The real voyage of discovery consists not in seeking new landscapes, but in having new eyes."

- Marcel Proust
(Novelist and Essayist)

I. Resistance, Impediments, and Common Obstacles to Mindfulness

We all have moments when we feel overwhelmed by our thoughts and emotions. It's part of the human experience. We get caught up in worries about the future, regrets about the past, or frustrations with the present moment. We might snap at a loved one, lash out in anger, or retreat into resentment and isolation.

Often, these reactions seem to come out of nowhere, leaving us feeling confused and even ashamed. You are not alone if you have ever felt overwhelmed by thoughts and emotions. I could probably fill another book listing all the ways that I have resisted and been caught in my own stories and dramas, self-assertion, and self-centric antics—all of which have served as my own impediments to any kind of mindful approach. But what if there's more to the story?

One of the biggest obstacles to mindfulness is our strong attachment to our thoughts, emotions, and sense of self.

We tend to identify with our thoughts ("I am a worrier," "I am strong," "I am no good," "I am very important," "I am so offended by...," etc.), and these powerful ties to our emotions become symbols and expressions of who we think we are ("I am angry!", "I am sad," "I feel betrayed...," and many more).

We invent, retell, and reaffirm our stories about who we are, defending them fiercely, even when they are so often the source of our emotional pain and anguish. Broadly speaking, these attachments often stem from unresolved deep-seated fears, past traumas (physical or emotional), or other insecurities.

These unchecked stories and our strong attachment to them can fuel a wide variety of negative reactions and behaviors, including explosive anger and rage, hurtful verbal outbursts, persistent blaming of others, and deep-seated resentments. They force us to vehemently defend our point of view and our beliefs at any cost, even if it means sacrificing our relationships or even our own happiness.

As the saying goes, "You are not really mad at what you think you're mad at." We might get angry at a coworker for a small mistake when the real source of our frustration is a larger work project. We might snap at our partner for dropping a plate when washing the dishes when we are actually feeling resentful about a bigger, unresolved issue in the relationship that has been festering for some time. We might feel frustrated and upset with a friend who canceled our plans when the real issue comes from our insecurity about our social life.

We cling to our notions of self-worth and self-importance as a means to stand out and actually "be somebody" in a world that believes "only the fittest survive."

About the Following List:

The lists that follow are simply "common human tendencies," and not personal flaws. If you find a trait on the list that resonates with your own life experience, remember that mindfulness isn't about eliminating these... Simply said, it is about your awareness of them so they exert less influence on your life decisions, both short-term and long term and your "life challenges" as well as your life's joys (e.g., navigating life changes, managing pain, reducing emotional upsets, enhancing life contentment, etc).

This attachment to self and ingrained patterns of thinking can manifest in many ways. Here are some common obstacles to practicing mindfulness, grouped by their nature:

1. ***Ego-Driven Attachments & Self-Image Focus:***
   (Obstacles rooted in maintaining a specific self-concept or sense of importance)

   ◇ The need to be special or important: Clinging to a sense of uniqueness or superiority.

   ◇ The need to be right (and make others wrong): Defending one's views rigidly, often dismissing others.

   ◇ Having "something to prove": Driven by a need for external validation or to overcome perceived shortcomings.

2. ***Overconfidence and Arrogance:***
   (An inflated sense of self-worth that prevents openness and learning.)

   ◇ Self-absorption: Excessive focus on one's own thoughts, feelings, and experiences, excluding awareness of others or the present moment.

   ◇ Insecurity: Underlying feelings of inadequacy that can paradoxically fuel ego defenses like arrogance or the need to be right.

   ◇ Savior complex: Defining oneself through the need to rescue or fix others, rather than allowing them their own journey.

◇ Unhelpful Mental Habits & Thinking Patterns: (Cognitive patterns that cloud awareness)

◇ Rigid thinking: Includes "my way or the highway" attitudes, insistence on things being a certain way, and concretized or inflexible views.

◇ Being judgmental: Constantly evaluating oneself, others, or situations negatively.

◇ Negative self-talk: Habitual inner criticism and putting oneself down.

3. *Overthinking and Worrying:*
(Getting lost in excessive analysis, rumination, or anxious thoughts about the past or the future.)

◇ Intolerance for differing opinions: Difficulty accepting or considering perspectives that challenge one's own.

◇ Paranoia: Pervasive distrust or suspicion that distorts perception.

◇ Personal agendas and ulterior motives: Approaching situations with hidden goals rather than open presence.

◇ Emotional Reactivity & Difficult States: (Being overwhelmed or driven by intense emotions)

◇ Fear: Allowing anxieties and fears to dominate awareness and decision-making.

◇ Anger: Frequent or easily triggered states of irritation, frustration, or rage.

◇ Resentment: Holding onto past grievances and bitterness.

◇ Excessive desire or craving: Strong attachment to wanting things (outcomes, possessions, sensations) to be different.

◇ Being overly dramatic: Amplifying emotional responses beyond the scale of the situation.

4. *Interpersonal & Behavioral Patterns:*

(Actions and ways of relating that hinder mindfulness)

◇ Restlessness (being overly talkative or fidgety): Physical or verbal agitation that makes stillness difficult.

◇ Being "mean-spirited" or belittling others: Acting out of negativity or a desire to diminish others.

◇ Deceitfulness: Lack of honesty with oneself or others.

◇ Predatory mindset: Viewing interactions as opportunities to exploit or gain advantage over others.

◇ Being an enabler: Supporting unhealthy patterns in others, often avoiding direct confrontation or presence with the difficulty.

◇ Addictions: Compulsive behaviors used to avoid discomfort or escape the present moment.

5. *Resistance & Disengagement:*

(Avoiding or refusing to engage with present reality)

◇ Non-acceptance of circumstances: Resisting or fighting against "what is."

◇ Boredom: Difficulty finding interest or engagement in the present moment.

◇ Disinterest or apathy: Lack of curiosity or care towards one's inner or outer experience.

Mindfulness offers a way to shift these perspectives. By cultivating a gentle awareness, an open kindness, non-biased full-hearted acceptance, with a relaxed child-like wonder, we can begin to loosen our grip on these attachments. We can learn to witness our thoughts and emotions without getting carried away, acknowledge our feelings without negative self-talk or harsh judgment, we can approach ourselves and others with naturally-arising understanding and compassion. These skills, explored in detail throughout this book, help us understand the deeper roots of our reactions and respond to life's challenges with greater wisdom, ease, and insight.

Mindfulness can be an antidote, a reset, a timeout for our challenging emotional states. It is a tool to savor life's joys more deeply, a lifestyle if we choose, an on-demand problem diffuser, a situation de-escalation tool, and a balm for our burning emotions. There are no physical impediments to mindfulness, whether it is a body with limitation, illness, injury, or deformity... the actual impediments to mindfulness arise through our thinking which informs our behaviors, our reactions, and our responses to life's challenges. The degree to which mindfulness is resisted is in direct proportion to the intensity, fervor, and attachment to the behaviors and characteristics that run counter to a mindful approach.

These obstacles are quite common which means we are not alone on this adventure. Mindfulness is a journey, not a destination. By taking the first steps toward gently relaxing into an open, receptive, and spacious awareness, you're already on the path to greater self-understanding, life contentment, and ease.

Next Up: Mindfulness Misconceptions—The Hype & Hyperbole

While mindfulness has become a popular topic that gets a lot of media attention these days, we have found there to be an abundance of misunderstandings and misconceptions.

II. Mindfulness Misconceptions: Our Perspectives

Even if you have a solid understanding of mindfulness, I want to point out that my approach, grounded in decades of experience helping people like you discover the joys and benefits of mindfulness, differs a bit from "traditional mindfulness" presentations in five key ways:

- Mindfulness should be adaptable, accessible, and easy to use.

- Explanations should be free of jargon, dogma, formality, and clinician-speak.

- Keep it relevant, addressing all of life, including challenges and the joyous side of life.

- Set aside all "should dos" and "must-dos," and prescriptive practice-oriented instructions.

- Showcase how mindfulness can be a relevant Life Tool for anyone, no matter their life path, faith, or social or cultural background or preference.

And it is this "different perspective" that informs and colors how we address the "misconceptions" we list below.

So don't be too surprised if some of our answers offer a slightly different and nuanced insight, that is fresh, friendly, and a more accessible take on mindfulness, especially for those navigating their later years and looking to give mindfulness some consideration, and even a try.

Mindfulness Misconceptions: Our In-Depth Review

The following extensive list of common mindfulness misconceptions covers a wide range of misunderstandings, from practical concerns about time commitment and technique to deeper questions about the nature of mindfulness itself.

I encourage you to browse through this list, even if you think you already understand mindfulness. We hope the following information helps you along your mindfulness journey. Let's dive in!

---

1) Misunderstandings About the Nature of Mindfulness

Mindfulness is difficult.

• I hear this quite a bit. And while mindfulness could be made difficult by the application of strict rules and prescriptive practice outlines, our approach is more life-inclusive and supportive, and it's a skill that can be easily learned and implemented by anyone at any time. It's not about achieving a certain level of proficiency, or reaching a special state of mind; it's about releasing our grasp of the burning coals that agitate our minds and emotions, and simply paying attention to the present moment, with gentle acceptance and calm. And while it's not difficult, like any life skill, a little bit of intentional effort and a willingness to explore pay dividends far beyond the small investment.

Is Mindfulness is about emptying my mind completely?

• Ah, the "empty mind" concern! This is a common misconception. Many people think that mindfulness is about stopping thoughts altogether, but that's not the case. In fact, having a busy mind is a perfect place to start. Think of your thoughts like waves in the ocean— they're always moving, getting swept along by the wind, rising, and falling. Mindfulness isn't about stopping the waves; it's about learning to surf them. It's about noticing your thoughts without getting swept away by them. It's about recognizing that having an "out of control mind" is OK and that you can start right where you are. Did you know that recent research shows compelling trends that seem to show that mindfulness techniques help to calm the mind by strengthening areas of the brain associated with mental focus.

Is Mindfulness Just a Trendy Form of Relaxation?

• "Trendy"? That sounds fun! And while some might present mindfulness as a new and trendy thing, its roots are as old as our DNA. Yes, relaxation can be an immediate benefit, but thinking of mindfulness as just relaxation is like saying a wheel is only for cars—it's capable of so much more. While relaxation focuses on calming the body and mind (which is great!), mindfulness goes deeper. It's about cultivating awareness and acceptance of all our experiences, both pleasant and unpleasant. Think of it this way: relaxation is like taking a break from the waves crashing on the shore, while mindfulness is learning to surf them. It's about developing a deeper understanding of how our minds work and how we can face and respond to life's challenges in ways that are better for us and the people we share our lives with. And science backs this up—studies show that mindfulness can actually change the structure and function of the brain in positive ways, effects that go far beyond simple relaxation and self-improvement.

Mindfulness is about avoiding difficult emotions.

• Mindfulness is about avoiding difficult emotions. That's a very common misunderstanding. Our approach to mindfulness isn't about suppressing or ignoring feelings. It's about developing a healthier relationship with them. It's about noticing emotions as they arise, acknowledging them with a calm acceptance, without bias, and looking at how they affect you, physically and mentally. This supports and informs your choices for responding while cooling the flames of intense emotions, rather than being swept up or controlled by them. It's about meeting and engaging with your emotions in a way that supports your overall well-being and the relationships with the people in your life.

Will Mindfulness will help me to eliminate all of my negative emotions?

• This is a question many people have, and the answer is a nuanced one. While mindfulness can be incredibly helpful in managing difficult emotions, it's not about eliminating them entirely. Experiencing a full range of emotions, including negative ones, is a natural part of being human. Mindfulness helps us work with those feelings in a healthier way by actively observing them without judgment and avoiding unhelpful reactive patterns. It's not about becoming an empty-headed, thoughtless, non-emotive robot; it's about becoming more aware of what it means to be human and embracing that humanity. It's about facing your feelings with greater kindness and self-compassion.

Mindfulness means I should never express my emotions.

• Mindfulness means I should never express my emotions. This is a big misconception. Mindfulness isn't about suppressing or bottling up your feelings. It's about experiencing and choosing how to respond to all your feelings, whether that means sharing them in appropriate and healthy ways, or simply being mindful of the emotional ebb and flow without sharing—no longer a slave to unchecked reactivity.

Mindfulness is just another kind of meditation.

• Mindfulness is just another kind of meditation. While this is an understandable interpretation, it's definitely not true. While mindfulness can be practiced during meditation, it's not limited to formal meditation practices. The approach I present emphasizes mindfulness as a way of engaging with the present moment in any activity, whether it's meditation, walking, eating, or simply noticing your breath. It's a skill that can be cultivated and applied to all aspects of life, a tool to enrich any activity.

Would mindfulness make me selfish?

• OK... It's easy to see how this is a common perspective, so let's unpack this a bit. Some people worry that focusing on one's experiences is inherently being self-absorbed or selfish. However, the approach I outline emphasizes that mindfulness, through both "self-focus" as a tool of self-inquiry, can actually improve our relationships. By cultivating a self-awareness that is "emotionally aware," it leads quite naturally to emotional regulation, allowing for a more accepting, empathetic, and compassionate perspective—qualities that strengthen connections with others. So yes, mindfulness is about "understanding yourself better," but only as a tool to help you relate to the world in more positive and insightful ways. Mindfulness is a tool to engage with yourself in a way that allows for deeper and more meaningful engagement with others and, over time, calms our inflammatory thinking, negative self-talk, our reactive responses.

Mindfulness means being passive.

• Mindfulness means being passive. Passive?! What!? Couldn't be further from the truth! My approach emphasizes that mindfulness is not about being passive or disengaged from life, or like someone who is getting steamrolled by life. It's about being actively engaged with the present moment. It's about paying attention to your thoughts, feelings, and sensations in the spirit of curious and gentle self-inquiry and a fully open and receptive awareness. AND It's about allowing conscious choices to arise rather than being burdened with automatic responses, fear, or negative self-talk when facing life's challenges. Mindfulness is a powerful Life Tool that throws "passivity" out the window and supports you in your efforts to live richer, more intentional and satisfying life, fully engaged and ready to go!

Mindfulness is boring.

• Mindfulness is boring. Ha! That's a good one! If you are bored with mindfulness then you aren't paying attention! This book's approach emphasizes that mindfulness can be anything but boring! It's about discovering and then rediscovering the richness of life in all its splendor, from the simple pleasures of a warm beverage, the astounding kaleidoscopic world around us, the complex inner tapestry of our thoughts and emotions. It's about engaging all this with a raw curiosity and receptivity, it's discovering joy and meaning everywhere. It's about bringing a sense of wonder, awe, and appreciation to everything you do. Mindfulness is literally a power tool that transforms "boring" into "beautiful," amazing, enjoyable, and rich. Even life's challenges take on a new dimension that is far beyond the boundaries of boring!

Mindfulness is about achieving a special state.

• Special State? Nope, not here! We are working with "what is" and not changing anything. And I am certainly not saying "you have to achieve a certain mental state" to be effective, or that you need to focus on some distant nebulous special achievement. We are simply grounded in the present, just as it is, without trying to change it, alter it, purify it, embellish it, sugarcoat it, or escape from it. It's so simple really... Just "pay attention" to your inner world (thoughts, feelings, and sensations) and your outer world (with all your senses) without adding elaborations, embellishments, drama, or anything at all. Just notice, then choose, act, and respond in ways that are meaningful and aligned with your values. It's not about seeking a special state; it's about diving in, facing challenges head-on, and also appreciating the incredible richness of life in all its aspects.

Mindfulness is the same as positive thinking.

• Mindfulness is the same as positive thinking. "Positive Thinking" is definitely not a bad thing... but it is not what mindfulness is about. And while mindfulness can contribute to a more positive outlook, the idea of choosing or forcing positive thoughts is antithetical to a mindfulness approach. When engaged with mindfulness and a "thought focus" is what is going on, it's just "observing and experiencing your thoughts" as they are, positive or negative or something in-between, without bias or rejection or any effort to change or shift them. Just fleeting mental events, passing like clouds. And of course, it's OK to "shift your thinking" as it may naturally occur to you, but the key thing is developing a relaxed awareness that embraces all thoughts (and feelings), without getting carried away by them. Mindfulness is about unelaborated awareness, and if needed or appropriate, making changes or taking action as we deem necessary. We are not promoting a magical world of "positive wishing", but rather a responsible response to life as it unfolds.

Mindfulness is about controlling my thoughts.

• Mindfulness is about controlling my thoughts. It would be quite a feat to be able to "control" our thoughts on demand. But the truth of the matter is that mindfulness is far more relaxed than that. A mindful approach "gently allows thoughts" to come and go, no matter their shape or intensity, rather than trying to employ some kind of mind control. Thoughts, as you likely know, are as much a part of our experience as DNA is of our cells. So, controlling thoughts, from the mindfulness perspective, is not particularly helpful. That's not to say we can't recognize thoughts that don't serve us or misrepresent how we see ourselves. We can shift things as needed. But the important point is that a mindful approach to thoughts incorporates non-biased acceptance and a gentle spirit of curious self-inquiry. By noticing thoughts, and eventually recognizing our thought patterns and thinking habits, we become empowered. Now our thoughts have loosened their grip, allowing us to adjust and tune our mental landscape simply releasing thoughts that no longer serve us. It's about skillfully riding the waves of thought—not trying to control them.

---

2) *Misunderstandings About the Difficulty/ Effort of Mindfulness*

Mindfulness is too strenuous.

• Mindfulness is too strenuous. Another good one! Not as common a misconception as some on the list, but it is worthy of addressing. The idea of "strenuous" implies great effort, and this is not the path of mindfulness. I emphasize the idea that mindfulness is an everyday, nothing-special, easy-to-use life tool, much like driving a car or enjoying a meal. It's easily woven into the fabric of everyday life and requires no intense physical exertion, awkward contortions, or even long periods of furrowed-brow focus. Notice the rhythm of your breath, the weight of your feet on the ground, the clatter in the kitchen, and even the hustle and bustle of a busy life... Just be "you" and be natural and gently nudge your awareness to whatever you're doing, in a way that feels natural, comfortable, and convenient for you.

Mindfulness requires too much concentration.

• Mindfulness requires too much concentration. Oh my, forced concentration? Ouch! If mindfulness required forced concentration, I would be off playing hooky whenever I could! But seriously, we do need to honestly address this. The idea of forced "concentration," implies "the achievement of some far-off obtainable goal," which is counter to the idea we present, "there is nothing to achieve," so forced concentration is not needed. My approach is a relaxed one, a soft and gentle nudge toward simply "noticing" our world. This includes the internal world of thoughts, feelings, and sensations, as well as the external world. It's a relaxed and open-to-all-of-life approach, where we meet and navigate life's meandering ups and downs with authenticity and sincerity. Nothing is forced, nothing is added—we simply meet life as it is, head-on with open, unbiased receptivity, adjusting our course as needed. It's also important to state that whatever degree of present-moment awareness you bring to bear is fine. Whether it's an as-needed reset when life throws you a curve-ball, or an intentional moment or two to simply savor life—just come as you are. Leave the "concentration" to the meditation experts while we enjoy the natural ebb and flow of our life.

Mindfulness is something I have to do perfectly.

• Mindfulness is something I have to do perfectly. If only! Truth be told, mindfulness is quite messy. Let me explain... Mindfulness is just "living life"... nothing special to do, no "perfect way of doing it." And just like life, which can be oh-so-messy and chaotic, mindfulness is just going along for the ride! Life and mindfulness are kind of like a carnival ride... a dazzling display of lights and sounds filling all your senses while you simply take it all in. But it's more than just going along for a ride... it's being "present" and noticing when thoughts or emotions are hijacking your joy or expression. We just let the world in and respond as we need to in ways that align with our needs, safety, and personality, all through the lens of present-moment awareness. So relax, and don't worry about "doing it right"—just have some fun, and remember that mindfulness is a tool that can both help you navigate life challenges, but also savor the ride!

I'm not good at meditating, so I can't be mindful.

• This is another very common misconception. The approach in this book isn't about teaching specific meditation techniques or improving or evaluating your meditation skills. While mindfulness can be practiced during meditation, our focus is on direct awareness—a present-moment awareness that is fully engaged in every aspect of life and not detached from it in any way—not as a formal practice, but as a life tool to help us break the patterns of habitual thinking, automated responses, and negative self-talk. Regardless of your meditation skills or lack thereof, you can definitely enjoy mindfulness! Walking, eating, listening to music, or even doing everyday tasks like washing dishes, and of course, all our emotions and thoughts, they are all part of the mindfulness playground. It's about bringing our attention to the present moment, whatever we're doing, whether it's for a few moments, a few minutes, day after day, or even a few times a week.

3) Misunderstandings About the Time Commitment of Mindfulness

Does Mindfulness Mean I Have to Sit Still for Hours?

• Absolutely not and who says you have to? Mindfulness isn't about forcing yourself into uncomfortable positions for a long time. When you engage with mindful approaches, we encourage you to use the techniques that you are drawn to and engage them in a way that is comfortable for you. Standing, lying down, walking, swaying, yoga, or even doing everyday tasks like washing dishes or even going to the gym, are all equally wonderful options for you to explore a mindful approach. The key is to bring your attention to the present moment, whatever you're doing. So, if you're someone who's always on the go or even limited in your abilities, don't worry—mindfulness still fits into your life in the way best suited for you.

Does mindfulness take a long time to do?

• It might, but only if you approach it from the perspective of it being "a formal practice" (which is fine, but not what we encourage). Our approach, in essence, is this; One moment of awareness is enough! And while that may seem a simplistic definition, it really does embody our presentation and approach. Imagine this: You, fully relaxed in the moment, with a wide-open, non-agenda receptive awareness. Release, even if only for a moment, any interpretative or reactive worldview. Just let the moment shine through—without the mental filters, the bias, the self-talk. Wouldn't that be enough?

How long does it take to get good at Mindfulness?

• It's a common question and concern and the answers range from "No time at all!" to "a lifetime". Here's why; most people believe that to get benefit from "techniques," mindfulness or otherwise, you have to first attain a certain level of proficiency which "takes time." In the end, it all comes down to your ability to "just notice" without getting caught up in our personal stories, bias, agenda, drama, and world view. From the mindfulness perspective, the more we cling and grasp to strongly held ideas of self and our stories, or ideas of "getting good at mindfulness," the more elusive the benefits will be. So we encourage a relaxed approach that is not focused on a nebulous goal, but rather a very relaxed gentle approach that settles into whatever is in our sphere of perception, whether it's thoughts, emotions, bodily sensations, or the myriad perceptions of the world around us.

I don't have time for mindfulness... Doesn't mindfulness take too long?

• Not at all! Mindfulness can fit into even the busiest schedules. Even a few short breaths, a few mindful moments of appreciation, or even a mini-dedicated mindful lunchtime bite or two can make a difference in your day. Rattled during your commute? Take a breath! Washing dishes? Enjoy the warm water! Taking a walk?

Enjoy the sounds! It's not about finding hours to dedicate to a formal practice; we are simply inviting you to gently weave mindfulness into the fabric of your daily life.

---

4) *Misunderstandings About the Benefits/ Expectations of Mindfulness*

Will Mindfulness Instantly Solve All My Problems?

• If only! Mindfulness isn't a magic wand that instantly erases all our problems. It's more of a skill, like learning a new language or playing a musical instrument. But the beauty of it is that many of the benefits can be reaped immediately! Think of it: calming down in the moment, reducing overwhelm in the moment, reducing anger in the moment—mindfulness provides a fantastic way to simply "reset" our upset or internal dialogues right now. While the long-term benefits and deeper results may take more time and consistent effort, don't think you can't experience some immediate relief and positive change. And, like with all skills, regular use helps us develop greater skills. Skills that can help us to regulate our emotions more effectively and respond to life's challenges with more balance, resilience, and ease. As my wife is fond of saying, "It's about progress, not perfection," and I couldn't agree more!

Will mindfulness instantly eliminate all negative emotions?

• We might wish this were true! While mindfulness can be very helpful in managing difficult emotions, it's definitely not a magic pill or a cure-all. It's more like a gentle, consistent approach that takes time and effort to develop. You'll still experience a full range of emotions. (Feeling sad, angry, or anxious is part of the human experience. Mindfulness helps us work with those feelings in a healthier way.)

Is mindfulness a quick fix?

• Mindfulness is a quick fix. If only! While mindfulness can offer moments of immediate relief and insight, it's not a magic bullet that instantly solves all our problems. We frame mindfulness as "tools for life"... tools that range from the "faster" (temporary relief when facing life challenges, to a more uplifting "joyful appreciation"), to longer-lasting life support tools. And while all are "easy to use," just like mechanics' tools, the benefit is gained through using them. Consider these three levels of mindfulness engagement:

◊ Use it on-demand and as-needed at the level you are comfortable with, using the simplest tools (one or two short breaths, simple movement).

◊ Engage with it as part of your day or week, incorporating some longer techniques for relaxation or calming emotional upset.

◇ Integrate mindfulness into your life as a long-term tool to help shift challenging emotions, mental patterns, or habitual behaviors.

• No matter how you choose to approach mindfulness, we honor your choice and believe it is a useful tool at any level of engagement.

Is mindfulness a substitute for therapy?

• Absolutely not. While mindfulness can be incredibly beneficial for mental and emotional well-being, it's not a replacement for professional therapy. Therapy provides a safe and supportive space to explore deep-seated issues, process trauma, and work through complex emotional challenges with a trained professional. And while mindfulness can be a valuable complement to therapy, enhancing self-awareness and emotional regulation, it shouldn't be considered a substitute for professional mental health care.

• **If you're struggling with significant mental or emotional challenges, we encourage you to seek the guidance of a qualified therapist.** They can provide the support and expertise you need to navigate your journey toward healing and well-being, and can help you understand the root causes of your challenges, develop coping mechanisms, and learn to re-frame negative or self-limiting thoughts. *(Mindfulness can support this process by enhancing your awareness of these thoughts as they arise, allowing you to bring that awareness to your therapy sessions.)*

Is mindfulness is a substitute for medical care (Rx, pain management)?

• Let's be 100% clear, mindfulness is NOT a replacement for professional medical care for illness or injury, psychiatric care, and any follow-up recommendations including prescription medications, pain management programs, or other medical treatments. Advanced care practitioners can accurately diagnose your condition, recommend appropriate treatments, and provide the medical expertise you need. (If you are experiencing physical pain, illness, or injury, it's essential to seek the guidance of a qualified medical professional or call 911 if it is an actual emergency)

• While mindfulness is not a healer in the "faith-healing" sense, research suggests that mindfulness techniques can play a supporting role in the healing process by calming the nervous system, easing anxiety, and reducing body tension. The consensus is that mindfulness can create a more conducive environment for our own healing and recovery process. Many spiritual traditions have also recognized the connection between mental and emotional well-being and physical health, incorporating practices like meditation and focused attention in their approaches to address illness and injury. However, it's crucial to emphasize that mindfulness should not be used as a substitute for evidence-based medical treatments. Instead, think of it as a valuable complement to professional medical care, supporting your overall well-being as you heal. It's about working with the medical team, not replacing them.

Will mindfulness take away my grief?

• The simple answer is no. Mindfulness is not a magic eraser that can stop, eliminate, or end grieving, nor can it replace the complex emotional process of mourning. Grief, as uncomfortable as it is, is a natural and deeply personal process—one that must be honored.

• However, mindfulness can provide valuable support during the grieving process, helping you navigate the intense emotions that arise, including sadness, anger, confusion, and loneliness. The mindfulness tools and techniques we present can help smooth the sharp edges of grief, ease emotional pain and anguish, and calm the turbulent thoughts that often accompany loss. Mindfulness can create a safe space to fully experience your grief. It can help you avoid being carried away by emotional turbulence and churning thoughts, allowing emotions to flow and naturally run their course.

• Remember, mindfulness is not a quick fix for grief, nor is it an escape mechanism to hide from raw emotions. It's a tool for developing a gentler, kinder relationship with yourself and your emotions, allowing you to move through the grieving process with clarity, ease, and resilience.

Isn't mindfulness is just another way for both young and old people to avoid dealing with difficult emotions?

• Not quite! While relaxation can be a welcome side effect of mindfulness, it's not the primary goal. Mindfulness is about cultivating present-moment awareness and non-judgmental observation of your emotions, which can have deeper benefits for emotional regulation and overall well-being. *(It's not about escaping your feelings or pretending they don't exist; it's about developing a new, healthier way of relating to your inner emotional world. It's about facing your feelings with greater kindness and compassion.)*

Does mindfulness mean you should never express your emotions>

• Definitely not! Sadly, this notion is more common than you might think, so let's address it head-on. Mindfulness is not about suppressing or denying your emotions (or even your thoughts), nor is it about becoming emotionally detached, robotic, or emotionally distant. Quite the opposite! Mindfulness is about cultivating a deeper awareness of all your emotions—happy, painful, and everything in between. It's about recognizing and acknowledging your feelings without self-criticism, self-judgment, or negative self-talk, allowing yourself to experience your full spectrum of emotions.

• In fact, mindfulness can actually enhance your ability to experience your feelings fully and express them in healthy and non-blaming ways. By exploring your inner emotional landscape through mindfulness tools and techniques, you gain greater sensitivity, awareness, and insight into what you're feeling and why. This empowers you to communicate your emotions more effectively, with greater clarity and authenticity, allowing you to choose how you want to respond rather than being controlled by them.

---

5) Misunderstandings About the Impact of Mindfulness on Personal Identity/Lifestyle

Mindfulness is about becoming a different person.

• No way... "You" will still be you! That said, mindfulness may shift the ideas or perceptions you have about yourself. If you tend to get caught up in your "stories" or personal dramas, are in a constant state of agitation or anxiety, engage in a lot of negative self-talk, express a lot of anger, are emotionally reactive, or feel overly burdened by life's challenges, mindfulness can be a life choice and tool that can ease these experiences.

Do I have to give up my sense of self?

• Definitely not. Your sense of self will continue to be your primary reference point when working with your experiences and when relating to the world around you. Your uniqueness is something that has value and is something to honor and celebrate. That said, your experience of "you" may shift in some ways, such as how you feel about yourself, how you see and relate to others, how you experience your emotions and thoughts, your relationship to life challenges and upsets, and your overall sense of well-being.

Does mindfulness means I have to give up my favorite things or activities (coffee, TV, social activities, exercise, etc.)?

• No way! Mindfulness, as we present it, is a way of being present with all of life, just as it is. There is no need to give up anything at all. We encourage everyone to continue living their life in the way that suits them. The key is awareness. Mindfulness isn't about avoiding activities; it's about engaging with them more consciously. Take driving, for example. Mindful driving isn't about closing your eyes and meditating behind the wheel! It's about being fully present while driving—aware of your surroundings, your car's movements, the traffic flow, and your own emotional state. This heightened awareness can actually make you a safer and more attentive driver. It's about bringing the same quality of attention to all aspects of your life, whether it's enjoying a cup of coffee, watching TV, or spending time with loved ones.

Does mindfulness means I have to get up extra early every day?

• Not at all. There is no need to adjust your sleep patterns, engage in esoteric practices, conform to some strict protocol, or make any lifestyle changes at all. Get all the sleep you need or want. In fact, we think that lounging in bed for a minute or two with a mindful breath or two or three, before you pop up to engage your day is a great way to start the day.

---

6) Misunderstandings About the Compatibility of Mindfulness with Religion/Spirituality

Is Mindfulness Only for Religious or Spiritual People?

• While this may have been the case in the past, it is definitely no longer true. In our contemporary culture, mindfulness is used in many non-religious applications, such as mental health, pain management, and as a quality-of-life enhancer. It is also the subject of recent and ongoing medical research aimed at documenting and understanding the correlations between mind, health, and healing. In this book, our focus is on mindfulness as a practical tool for life enhancement—whether that is working with challenging emotions, runaway thoughts, health issues, or simply enriching our appreciation of life. Personally, I think that mindfulness is a fantastic tool for everyone, regardless of background, beliefs, physical limitations, or spiritual inclination.

Mindfulness is against my religious beliefs and will interfere with my ability to find emotional comfort in my faith:

- This is an interesting question that deserves a thoughtful explanation. In our current culture, mindfulness has become a mainstream secular activity, rooted in scientific research, and is seen by many as a technique that can complement and integrate with any belief system. As a tool, mindfulness is simple an expression of your inner calm and naturally aware state. While there is much discussion about mindfulness as a potential tool or technique, both theistic perspectives or a more universal, holistic approach, the tools and techniques that mindfulness offers, from our perspective, support the whole person—no matter their faith or religious practice. Many believe that mindfulness is a perfect complement to traditional prayer, faith-based contemplation, and meditation or visualization practices with the potential to deepen and enrich those practices. (Note: If you are in doubt, please consult with leaders in your faith-tradition that may offer additional insights.)

Do I have to become a Buddhist to practice mindfulness?

- Nope... Mindfulness is a life tool for anyone, regardless of faith or philosophy. Think of it this way: A Zen Master, a Rabbi, a car mechanic, and a child are all sitting together in a garden with rapt attention, watching a lizard climb across a stone wall. Each has their own life perspective, yet each is attentively watching the lizard. "Watching" is what mindfulness is... and that is something anyone can do, regardless of their faith or life perspective.

Does working with mindfulness mean I need to adopt a monastic lifestyle?

• Absolutely not! Mindfulness, as we present it, is a tool for enhancing your life as it is. It's not about adopting a new restrictive lifestyle and renouncing your current life, relationships, or beliefs. You certainly don't need to become a monk or nun, live in a monastery, or give up any aspects of your life that are meaningful, important, and joyous for you. Mindfulness is a simple approach that is just about meeting your life as it is with a gentle open awareness, and whatever experiences and situations that includes. It's about relaxing and meeting life head-on, not escaping from it. You can be a mindful parent, a mindful professional, a mindful partner, a mindful cook, and a mindful friend—mindfulness is just another way of living your life and enhancing the roles you already play.

7) *Misunderstandings About the Impact of Mindfulness on Relationships/Social Connections*

Is Mindfulness a solitary technique that must be done alone?

• Oddly enough, the answer is both yes and no. Here's what I mean. Yes, in the sense that there is a singular "you" experienced as "I, me, and mine." This triad of self-affirming references infuses our language, thinking, relationships, and social interactions. So, from that perspective, mindfulness is and can only ever be a solitary technique. But the "no" answer reveals the important relational aspect of mindfulness. Here, "relationship" refers to the entirety of the world we interact with—people, things, situations, challenges, etc.—which constitute the fertile ground of our mindfulness explorations. One way to think about this is that mindfulness, a solitary technique, thrives in the panoramic expanse of everything and everyone.

Does mindfulness means I have to give up my friendships and relationships?

• This couldn't be further from the truth. All relationships—intimate, friendships, social, acquaintances, professional, etc.—are important in the context of mindfulness. They all present unique experiences and opportunities to explore and express our inner landscape (feelings, thoughts, and emotions), providing a rich tapestry that gives context to our lives, and allows us to shape and embody the life we choose.

Will mindfulness make me distant from my loved ones?

• Only if you misunderstand our presentation of mindfulness as a Life Tool. From my perspective, mindfulness is an all-inclusive approach, capable of engaging any situation or life experience, from exuberant joy to upsetting challenges. Mindfulness delivers the greatest benefit when it fully engages with all of life, including our closest relationships. Limiting or excluding anything from the mindfulness journey is like going for a walk on a beautiful spring day while wearing a blindfold and earplugs. The entire spectrum of life is the domain of mindfulness, so please don't think you have to give anything up or alter your life or relationships in any way in order to explore mindfulness.

---

8) Misunderstandings About the Practical Concerns of Mindfulness

Do I need to dedicate a lot of time to mindfulness?

• I say, absolutely not! As we've noted before, even one moment of awareness is enough. (See Chapter 3, "The Story Behind These Mindful Moments," for more on this.) This simple definition captures the essence of our approach. Imagine: You, fully relaxed in your favorite place, with a wide-open, no-agenda, receptive awareness. Interpretive thoughts released, each moment a panoramic, kaleidoscopic awareness—without mental filters, bias, or self-talk. Wouldn't that be enough?

Does Mindfulness Require Special Equipment or a Special Place?

• Nope! You don't need fancy cushions, incense, or a quiet retreat in the mountains to engage with mindfulness techniques. They can be used anywhere, anytime—at home, in your car, or even while waiting in line at the grocery store. It's about bringing your attention to the here and now, wherever you are—a simple mindful breath while waiting for the kettle to boil or noticing the sensations as you wash your hands is all it takes.

Does mindfulness require an in-person teacher?

• Simply put, no. While in-person instruction can be helpful, many outstanding resources on mindfulness are available, including books, online videos, podcasts, online support groups, and websites. Even private and small group "mindfulness coaching" is available via live video conferencing.

Is there a mindfulness certification?

• Surprisingly, yes! Colleges, non-profit organizations, and private businesses offer "mindfulness certificates." Some programs are designed for those who want to teach mindfulness, while others focus on personal development. A simple online search for "mindfulness certification programs" will provide more information.

Do I need to keep a mindfulness journal?

• No, keeping a journal is not a requirement for working with mindfulness techniques. That said, a journal can be a useful tool when you are either navigating life challenges or simply want to track your progress or experiences as you explore mindfulness strategies.

I have heard mindfulness is not safe when driving. Is that true?

• There are two perspectives on this. Our approach is that mindfulness isn't about avoiding activities; it's about engaging with them more consciously, with greater focus and attention—and this includes driving. Mindful driving means being fully aware of your surroundings, your car's movements, traffic flow, safety, road conditions, and your emotional state. We believe that mindful driving is safe driving. Of course, we strongly discourage any kind of "meditation" or closing your eyes while behind the wheel!

9) *Misunderstandings About Who Can Benefit from Mindfulness*

Am I Too Old to Start Working With Mindfulness?

• Absolutely not! Because mindfulness is so adaptable and flexible, it can be tailored to fit your specific needs, inclinations, and abilities. Whether you prefer longer periods of focused attention, shorter moments of mindful awareness, or even a quick pause and reset, mindfulness can work for you. And here's why it's never too late to learn new skills. Our brains possess an amazing capacity to change and adapt throughout our lives—something now known as neuroplasticity. Just as we can create new pathways in a garden to connect different areas, our brains can form new neural pathways and connections at any age. This makes mindfulness an easy-to-adopt, life-enhancing tool for any stage of life. In fact, mindfulness can be particularly helpful for seniors, providing a proven framework for meeting and managing common age-related challenges, including anxiety reduction, improved sleep, enhanced cognitive function, greater emotional well-being, and increased life satisfaction.

Isn't mindfulness is only for young people?

• That's simply not true. Mindfulness can easily be adapted to suit any age, inclination, physical condition, or ability. It doesn't require any special youthful mental agility—just a willingness to try. Whether we're navigating difficult emotions, exploring personal growth, or seeking a bit more joy in life, mindfulness is about meeting ourselves where we are, regardless of age, health, personality, or background. It's never too late to learn a new life skill that can help us navigate life's challenges or add another level of richness to our life's enjoyment. Think of it as a little life boost.

Am I too old to learn new ways of managing my emotions?

• Not at all! It's never too late to learn new skills, especially those related to our emotions and feelings. As we've discussed, our brains possess an amazing capacity to change and adapt throughout our lives—a capacity known as neuroplasticity. And this ability isn't limited to learning new songs or improving chess strategies; it also allows us to learn how to understand and effectively work with our emotions at any age. Many seniors have found mindfulness particularly helpful for navigating the myriad emotional challenges that arise from life's inevitable ups and downs. Mindfulness offers tools that help us understand our emotions, calm our upsets, and reset our overreactions—key benefits for emotional well-being.

Isn't mindfulness is only for people who are stressed or anxious?

• While it might seem that way, consider the vast range of emotions we experience—from fleeting wisps to immovable icebergs. Mindfulness is a versatile tool that can benefit everyone, regardless of their emotional state. Yes, it can be particularly helpful for managing stress and anxiety, but it can also enhance self-care, self-awareness, mental focus, and overall life enjoyment. (It's much more than just a tool for managing problems like stress and anxiety; it's a way to reimagine, reshape, and re-embrace your life—your whole life!)

Is Mindfulness Just for Super Calm People?

• Absolutely not! Mindfulness isn't just for monks meditating in caves or people who are naturally calm and serene. It's for everyone—including those of us who feel stressed, anxious, or even a little bit grumpy sometimes. In fact, those who struggle with difficult emotions may find mindfulness especially helpful. While it may be a new skill to learn—you don't have to be an expert to start or get some benefit. Just a simple engagement with even the most basic techniques can help us to become calmer, more focused, and more resilient in the face of life's challenges or even discover a new level of richness in our lives.

Isn't Mindfulness only for certain personality types?

• That's simply not true. Mindfulness can be used by everyone, regardless of their personality, work status, age, or physical abilities. No matter if you're an introvert or an extrovert, a thinker or a feeler, or an action-oriented get-things-done sort of person, mindfulness can be tailored to fit your unique style and preferences. It's not about changing who you are; it's simply about bringing a gentle mindful focus to your life at whatever level you choose or are comfortable. It's a soft skill that can be learned and adopted by anyone who's willing to give it a try.

III. The History of Mindfulness

From Ancient Wisdom to Modern Practice: A Brief History of Mindfulness

The following historical overview of mindfulness is based on widely available information and general knowledge of contemplative traditions.

Mindfulness, the practice of present-moment awareness, has deep roots in various cultures and traditions across the globe. While the term "mindfulness" itself is relatively recent, the underlying principles of focused attention, non-judgmental observation, and acceptance have been explored and cultivated for centuries. Many traditions offer what we might call "near mindfulness" approaches, practices that share core similarities with mindfulness even if they use different terminology or contexts. As we explore this rich history, it's inspiring to realize that these practices, passed down through generations, are available to us today, offering valuable tools for navigating the challenges and opportunities of later life.

1. **Prehistory:**

   ◇ **Shamanistic traditions and indigenous practices worldwide** incorporate altered states of consciousness and present-moment awareness, often through rituals, nature connection, and focused intention. These practices laid the foundation for later codified contemplative traditions.

2. **Early Eastern Traditions:**

   ◇ **Hinduism (c. 1500-500 BCE):** Rooted in the Vedas, practices like dhyana (meditation) and vipassana (insight) emphasize introspection and detachment from thoughts. The Upanishads further elaborate on these concepts, focusing on the nature of self and reality.

   ◇ **Jainism:** Develops practices emphasizing non-violence, self-control, and mindfulness of thoughts, words, and actions to minimize harm and attain liberation.

   ◇ **Buddhism (c. 6th Century BCE):** Emerging from Hinduism, Buddhism systematizes mindfulness through the Satipatthana Sutta, outlining mindfulness of body, feelings, mind, and mental objects. Both monastic and lay practices are developed, laying the groundwork for many modern mindfulness techniques.

3. Other Religious Traditions (Near Mindfulness):

◇ **Judaism:** Jewish contemplative practices, such as Kavvanah (intention) in prayer and meditation on scripture, encourage mindfulness. The Kabbalah tradition involves meditative techniques for deeper spiritual insight.

◇ **Christianity:** Contemplative prayer, such as centering prayer and Lectio Divina, focuses on present-moment awareness and union with God. Monastic traditions, like those of the Desert Fathers, emphasize stillness and introspection. These practices resonate with many seniors who have a lifelong connection with Christian traditions.

◇ **Islam:** Sufism, the mystical branch of Islam, incorporates practices like dhikr (remembrance of God) through repetitive chanting and meditation, fostering mindfulness of the divine presence.

◇ **Quakerism:** The Quaker tradition emphasizes silent worship and inner reflection, cultivating mindfulness through stillness and attentive listening to the "inner light."

4. Western Philosophical Traditions:

◇ **Ancient Greece:** Philosophers such as Socrates, Plato, and Aristotle emphasize self-awareness and introspection as essential for ethical living.

◇ **Stoicism:** A Hellenistic philosophy emphasizing present-moment awareness, acceptance of what cannot be controlled, rational thought as paths to tranquility, and living in accordance with nature. (Stoicism, derived from the Greek stoa meaning "porch," was a philosophy emphasizing virtue, reason, and living in harmony with the natural order. Key figures like Marcus Aurelius and Seneca advocated for self-control, resilience, and accepting what we cannot change.) This focus on acceptance and non-judgment echoes the core principles of mindfulness, encouraging us to observe our thoughts and feelings without getting carried away by them.

5. **Indigenous Cultures (Near Mindfulness):**

◇ **Various indigenous cultures worldwide** have incorporated mindfulness-like practices, such as shamanistic journeying, nature meditation, and focused rituals, to connect with the natural world and promote healing. These practices often emphasize connection to the earth and the cycles of life, which can be a source of comfort and meaning for seniors.

6. **Modern Developments:**

◇ **20th Century:** Mindfulness gains traction in the West through Buddhist teachers like Thich Nhat Hanh and the development of secular mindfulness programs such as Mindfulness-Based Stress Reduction (MBSR) by Jon Kabat-Zinn in 1979.

◇ **New Age:** The New Age movement integrates mindfulness with various spiritual and self-help practices, often emphasizing personal growth and holistic well-being.

◇ **21st Century:** Mindfulness becomes increasingly mainstream, integrated into various fields, including healthcare, education, business, and sports. Scientific research continues to explore its benefits for mental and physical health.

Mindfulness has evolved and adapted over centuries, offering a rich tapestry of practices that can enhance our lives at any age. We encourage you to explore these various traditions further and discover which practices resonate most deeply with you.

(See Summary Timeline Graphic on the next page)

Mindfulness: A General Timeline

EARLY NEAR-MINDUFLNESS

Prehistory: Early shamanistic and indigenous practices emphasize altered states of consciousness and present-moment awareness.

c. 1500-500 BCE: Hinduism's Vedas introduce dhyana (meditation) and vipassana (insight).

c. 6th Century BCE: Buddhism systematizes mindfulness through the Satipatthana Sutta.

Ancient Greece: Philosophers like Socrates, Plato, and Aristotle emphasize self-awareness and introspection.

1st-7th Centuries CE: Contemplative traditions develop in Judaism, Christianity, and Islam.

Medieval Period: Contemplative practices are further elaborated in Eastern and Western religions.

19th Century: Western interest in Eastern spiritual traditions increases.

MODERN MINDUFLNESS

1966: Thich Nhat Hanh exiled from Vietnam due to his peace activism, traveling to the West to teach mindfulness and establish communities.

1979: Jon Kabat-Zinn develops Mindfulness-Based Stress Reduction (MBSR).

21st Century: Mindfulness becomes culturally mainstream and is integrated into various health programs/practices supported by scientific research.

"Mindfulness, at its heart,
is a deep relaxation of our thoughts
and emotions... an openness to the
kaleidoscopic arc of life."

Blair O'Neil
(Excerpted from "Mindfulness for Seniors")

Chapter 1

"Be Here Now!"
Ram Dass

"With the past, I have nothing to do;
nor with the future. I live now."

Ralph Waldo Emerson

"Life is here, right now...
All we have to do is show up.
And the present moment is our ticket in."

Blair O'Neil
(Author and founder of Mindfulness for Seniors)

CHAPTER LEVEL TABLE OF CONTENTS

Chapter 1: The Present Moment: A Path to Transformation

Chapter 1

The Present Moment:
The Pathless Path of Transformation

I: Arriving in the Present

You know, sometimes I think my middle name should have been "Worry-wort." Especially when I became a dad at 45—suddenly, I was juggling a new career, a beautiful new son, and a wife who was now a full-time mom. For that first year, my mind was a runaway train of worries, keeping me up at night and making my days pretty anxious, too. Looking back, I realize much of that anxiety stemmed from my mind replaying the same old "worry and woe" soundtrack. Thankfully, I had some good friends, a good therapist, and basic experience with mindfulness... each playing their part to help me navigate that challenging time. And now many years later, having lost many of those good friends along the way, and that therapist no longer in the picture, it is mindfulness that continues to help me navigate life's amazing but tumultuous seas.

Our Experience of Time

As we begin our journey together in this book, let's take a moment to consider time, because this helps explain why mindfulness is so effective. We THINK of time as having three distinct parts: past, present, and future. We have memories of the past, plans for the future, and then there's right now, the place from which our stories unfold. We also have many different ways of understanding time, from history books and family stories to scientific and spiritual perspectives. But here's the key: we can't actually go back to the past, and we can't jump ahead to the future. *Our only direct EXPERIENCE of time is this very moment. Right now.*

The Importance of This Moment:

So, if all we really have is this present moment of now, then "now" becomes pretty important, doesn't it? It's where we have the power to choose and navigate our lives. Think of it as the driver's seat of your life, where you can choose your destination and route. It's where we can start to truly notice what's happening, rather than simply thinking or reacting habitually. It's a place where we can make conscious choices about how we want to respond to situations. By focusing on the present, we begin to disengage from the autopilot-self and become more aware of what is actually happening in us and around us, freeing ourselves from the grip of old mental and emotional patterns. Plus, by focusing on the present we can begin to:

- Become more aware of our inner dialogue

- Recognize old patterns of thinking and feeling

- Experience more calm our day-to-day lives

- Effectively face stress, worry, and difficult emotions

- Develop a deeper understanding of ourselves

- Connect with others more authentically

Our Journey Begins:

In this book, I'll be introducing you to a lot of ideas, perhaps many of them new to you. We will be presenting both contemporary and time-honored mindfulness approaches—focusing on how you can gain the benefits of mindfulness just by using simple exercises. I will share and explain the basics as well as introduce some more in-depth approaches. But don't worry, everything we present is going to be done in a way that is flexible and adaptable to your unique needs.

It's no secret that as we age, we find our experience of life shifting in unexpected ways, and more often than not it seems, shifts that require a bit of adjustment and adaptation. In support of this and your needs, we are going spend a lot of time reviewing lots of easy-to-use and practical techniques for working with your thoughts, feelings, physical sensations, and how to meet life's challenges in a balanced and responsible way. Together, we will also be spending some time exploring the connections and interplay between our thinking, emotions, and bodies, and they all affect our personality, social communication, and our sense of self. And, of course, I will share ways you can easily apply mindfulness to any aspect of your life—from the joyful stuff to the more challenging situations.

There will also be a few short deeper dives into topics that can make a huge impact on the quality of our lives, like physical health challenges, pain and discomfort, emotional ups and downs, grief, loss, and navigating all the changes in one's life—all while exploring the other side of the coin, life contentment, gratitude, patience, and self-compassion.

In this first chapter:

Next up, I'll explore how our self-talk and mental habits (developed over the years), combined with our emotions and reactivity, influence how we experience—and sometimes avoid—the present moment. We're going to start by looking at something key—our internal mental chatter, that constant inner voice and then move on from there. Now that we've introduced the idea and tried to relay the importance of the present moment, we're ready to wade into the shallow end of the mindfulness pond and explore the inner workings of our minds, starting with our inner dialogue.

II. Understanding Our Inner Dialogue: The Voice in Our Head

You know, most of us have this constant inner narrative going on—a little voice chattering away inside our heads that only we can hear. It's our non-stop chatty companion, continually sharing their views through thick and thin. And while this inner voice often expresses simple preferences, like "Ooh, I like this!," or "I want that!," it also voices our dislikes with a firm "Nope, not a fan of this." And here's the important point to remember, we're constantly navigating our world based on our little internal voice that is forever expressing their likes and dislikes, while we oblige that voice by moving towards what feels good and away from what causes us displeasure, discomfort, and pain.

And it's this constant self-talk, developed over a lifetime, that takes on the role of perpetual background soundtrack, filtering and coloring everything we experience and influencing pretty much everything we think, say, decide, and do. It not only shapes how we see ourselves, but also how we see other people, and how we see and relate to the entire world around us.

It's important to understand that not all self-talk is negative and that we're not trying to eliminate it; instead, the goal, via mindfulness approaches, is to simply become more aware of it, which allows us to live from the space of choice rather than from mental patterns and repeating loops.

No matter what proficiency or skill we gain with mindfulness, the potential benefits make even the simplest techniques a worthy endeavor because of the potential for personal transformation.

Common Self-Talk Patterns

Let's explore some common kinds of self-talk, focusing on those that can be particularly challenging and formative. I've found it helpful to think about self-talk in terms of whether it's healthy or unhealthy, and whether we're conscious of it or not. While these aren't scientific categories, they can be useful in helping us understand how our inner dialogue operates.

The most challenging area where unhealthy self-talk operates is in the realm of "unconscious self-talk." Once we become aware of this using super-simple, short mindful explorations, the unhealthy self-talk patterns become increasingly clear. And that clarity allows us to choose other responses, something more in line with the "person we want to be," rather than the person who is living a life of automatic unconscious responses.

Here are a few examples of unhealthy self-talk:

- **"I want," "I need," "I must have":** This type of self-talk focuses on instant gratification and can lead to addictive behaviors, from substance abuse to less obvious forms like overspending or unhealthy eating habits. It can also lead to neglecting practical considerations like safety or resources.

• **Insistence on being right:** This "bull in a china shop" self-talk arises from a sense of self-importance and often involves judging, belittling, or dismissing others' perspectives. It creates a "my way or the highway" approach to life, which can harm or antagonize our personal, friendly, or workplace relationships.

• **Negative and fear-based thinking:** This type of self-talk is rooted in low self-esteem and often involves thoughts like "I can't do that," "I don't deserve that," "What will they think of me?," or "I'm not good enough." It can also involve catastrophizing, exaggerating potential negative consequences ("If I make a mistake, everything will fall apart"), or using "should" statements that create unrealistic expectations ("I should be able to handle this on my own"). This kind of thinking can rob us of creativity, joy, and contentment, leading to avoidance, isolation, and a reluctance to take responsibility.

As we said, often we're not even aware of this constant inner dialogue. It runs in the background and is so ingrained in our daily lives from an early age that not only have we become used to it, but we also identify with this voice to such a degree that we may even think "This is just how I am." And that is why it's important to understand and recognize this far-too-influential voice, that often runs more of our lives that we'd care to admit to.

Head's Up! Easy Exercise Ahead! A gentle reminder:

Don't stress... There are no right or wrong answers. This is simply an exploration to help you become more aware of your inner world.

Here's a simple exercise that can help you become more aware of your own self-talk:

Exercise: Exploring Your Self-Talk

• **Reflect:** Take a few minutes to reflect on your own inner dialogue. You can use a journal, a piece of paper, a note-taking app, or simply contemplate this.

• **Notice:** Pay attention to the types of thoughts that come up. Are they mostly positive or negative? Do you notice any recurring themes or patterns? Do you feel any body sensations such as a smile, or conversely, a heaviness on your shoulders or tightness or tension anywhere in your body?

• **Connect to Decisions:** Consider how your self-talk might be influencing your daily decisions or even major life choices in the past or present.

The Key Self-Talk Take-Away

Becoming aware of your unconscious, unhealthy self-talk is the first and most important step toward making positive changes. When we start to understand how these mental patterns are influencing our lives, we can begin to gently free ourselves from their grip and open ourselves up to a more positive, engaged, and fulfilling set of life experiences. In the next section, we'll dive deeper into self-talk as a set of mental habits and explore just how much these habits can impact the quality of our lives.

III. Understanding Our Mental Habits

Challenging Ideas Ahead:

Go slow with this next section. Consider the ramifications and whether or not this resonates for you. There are a lot of important concepts to consider.

How many times a day do you try something truly new? A new approach to a familiar problem? A new way of interacting with someone challenging? A new food? A new route to a familiar destination? A new genre of book?

If you're like most of us, the answer is probably "not very often." Many of our daily activities, problem-solving strategies, interactions, even our food choices and leisure activities, are variations on a theme—guided by repeated thoughts, which in turn lead to repeated choices, actions, and reactions.

Habitual Thoughts = Habitual Actions

Our habitual thoughts—those little inner dialogue friends— directly translate into habitual actions. These thoughts act as both inner angels and inner demons, subtly influencing our lives, often without our conscious awareness. The more we repeat these thoughts and actions, the stronger the connections in our brains become, making these patterns more automatic over time. This automatically drives our behaviors, creating well-worn paths (aka; recurring themes) in our lives.

But here's the key: when these habitual patterns go unchecked, these paths can lead to both comfortable grooves and undesirable outcomes—from simple discomfort to even danger, or simply choices that aren't in our best interest, no matter how reassuring or comfortable those repeated mental habits might feel. And as we age, these mental habits can become even more deeply ingrained and resistant to change.

Two main sources of our mental patterns:

• **Pain Avoidance:** Physical or emotional traumas can create powerful avoidance patterns. These patterns can range from subtle self-protective mechanisms to more extreme reactions like PTSD, emotional shutdown, isolation, anger, or abrasive personality traits. While not everyone experiences extreme trauma, we all experience some degree of it—the loss of a loved one, serious illness, financial setbacks, job loss, natural disasters, social exclusion, bullying, or harassment.

• **Pleasure/Arousal:** "Feel-good" scenarios can also create powerful patterns associated with our wants, desires, and pursuits. While pleasurable experiences might seem positive, the unchecked pursuit of pleasure can lead to self-destructive behaviors and damage relationships. Addiction, in its various forms (from substance abuse to more subtle addictions like an excessive need for success or specific outcomes), is a key example of this. These patterns can manifest as blaming, belittling others, anger responses, or even emotional manipulation in relationships.

External Influences on Our Thinking

It's also important to recognize that our mental habits can be influenced by external forces. Various ideologies, established belief systems, marketing campaigns, and other external messages often appeal to our desires for pleasure or our fears of pain to shape our beliefs and behaviors. These influences can be particularly powerful when they resonate with pre-existing patterns of thinking. By becoming more mindful of our own mental habits, we can also become more aware of how external messages might be influencing us, allowing us to consider our responses and reactions.

It's important to note that while some mental habits stem from trauma or addiction, everyone experiences these patterns in varying degrees. Even seemingly minor mental habits, if left unchecked, can still negatively impact our lives. Here are some common examples:

• **Over-generalization:** Drawing broad conclusions based on limited evidence.

- **Lazy Thinking:** Taking mental shortcuts and avoiding careful consideration of the facts.

- **Emotional Reasoning:** Letting emotions dictate our thinking rather than considering all the facts.

- **Catastrophizing/Jumping to Conclusions:** Automatically assuming the worst possible outcome.

- **"Should" Statements:** Holding ourselves to rigid rules about how we "should" or "shouldn't" act.

- **Personalization:** Taking personal responsibility for things outside our control.

- **All-or-Nothing Thinking:** Seeing things in black and white, with no middle ground.

- **Discounting the Positive/Focusing on the Negative:** Ignoring positive experiences and dwelling on negative ones.

- **Overthinking:** Analyzing things excessively to the point of inaction.

We now stand at a crossroads: we can continue to navigate life on autopilot, driven by our habitual thoughts and responses, or we can begin to become aware of them and work with them consciously. Mindfulness is a powerful tool for this process. While these patterns can feel deeply ingrained, it's important to remember that they are not fixed. With awareness and conscious effort, we can begin to shift these habits and create new, more beneficial ways of thinking. In the next section, we'll explore the close relationship between mental habits and our emotional habits.

IV. Navigating the Emotional Landscape

Caution: More Weighty Topics Ahead

Once again, go slow with this next section. Consider if anything applies to your situation. We believe the following ideas are important to consider.

The Difference Between Thoughts, Emotions, and Feelings: Before we dive into navigating the emotional landscape, it's helpful to clarify the subtle and potentially confusing differences between thoughts, emotions, and feelings, as these terms are often used interchangeably. In essence:

- **Thoughts are mental processes**—ideas, beliefs, interpretations, and so on. They are cognitive and can be consciously influenced.

- **Emotions are more complex**, involving physiological changes in the body, subjective experiences, and behavioral expressions. They are often triggered by our thoughts or by external events.

- **Feelings are our subjective experiences** or interpretations of those emotions—the conscious awareness of what we are experiencing in our bodies and minds.

For example, the thought "I might be late" could trigger the emotion of anxiety, which we then feel as worry, tension, or a knot in our stomach. Understanding these differences and subtle distinctions will be crucial as we explore how to work with our emotions more effectively.

The Dance of Thoughts and Emotions: The relationship between thoughts and emotions is complex—they're not always neatly separated, with one always coming before the other. Sometimes, our emotions react instantly to an event, almost before we even have time to think. Other times, it's our thoughts—how we interpret and make sense of things—that spark an emotional response. It's probably more accurate to think of them as constantly influencing each other, like a dynamic dance. For example, a sudden surprise might cause an immediate emotional reaction, while a more complicated situation might need some thought before we feel anything. Ultimately, whether thoughts or emotions come "first" isn't the main point—both play a big part in how we experience our world.

Common Human Experience and Integrated Approach: It's important to remember that feeling all sorts of emotions—even the tough ones—is just part of being human. Everyone experiences emotional ups and downs; there's nothing wrong with feeling sad, angry, or afraid.

When it comes to emotional well-being, taking an integrated approach is key. Mindfulness is a great tool, but it's most effective when combined with other healthy habits, like connecting with others, getting enough sleep, moving your body, spending time outdoors, and being mindful of what media you consume.

Working with Our Core Emotions:

Fear and Anger: Now, fear is something we all experience. It pops up when we sense a threat—whether it's a real danger or just something we imagine—to our safety, our health, or even just how we see ourselves. You might notice it as feelings of anxiety, worry, or even a full-blown panic attack. Physically, your heart might start racing, your breath might get shallow, and your muscles might tense up.

And here's the interesting thing: When we feel like we can't do anything about the threat, or when the fear just gets too overwhelming, it can often turn into anger. This anger can be directed at whatever we think is causing the problem, or even at ourselves. For instance, if you're worried about losing your independence, you might find yourself getting irritated with people who try to help, even though they mean well. It's like you're seeing their help as a reminder of what you're afraid of losing.

For seniors, these fears might be related to declining health, changes in physical abilities, concerns about finances, or worries about becoming a burden on family. These very real concerns can sometimes manifest as frustration or anger, even towards loved ones.

The Influence of Self-Talk and Thinking Habits on Fear/Anger: Our self-talk plays a crucial role here. Fearful self-talk, such as "I'm not strong enough to handle this," can amplify the fear, while angry self-talk, such as "This is unfair!" can justify the anger. Mindful self-talk, such as "It's okay to feel afraid, and I can choose how I respond," can help us manage these emotions more effectively. It's easy to get caught up in these feelings, a phenomenon known as cognitive fusion *(See definition inset below)*. We lose the ability to observe them objectively and become swept away by their intensity. Imagine trying to navigate a storm at sea while believing you are the storm.

Mindfulness is like finding a safe bank on the river's edge. A place to get out of the turbulent waters of our intense emotions.

By focusing on our breath and noticing the sensations in our body, we can begin to observe our fear and anger with more clarity. Simply naming the emotion—"I'm feeling afraid," or "I'm feeling angry"—can also help reduce its intensity.

Understanding this connection can help us recognize the underlying fear driving our anger and respond more constructively.

Understanding Cognitive Fusion:

Cognitive fusion happens when we buy into our thoughts and emotions as absolute truths, rather than recognizing them as passing mental events. We become so "fused" with them that we react as if they are completely real and accurate reflections of reality, even when they might not be. This can lead to increased emotional distress and impulsive reactions. Mindfulness helps us to defuse from our thoughts and feelings, creating a little space so we can choose how to respond rather than simply reacting automatically.

Sadness and Joy: Sadness and joy, while they might seem like total opposites, are actually both really important parts of being human. Sadness usually shows up when we experience a loss, a disappointment, or when we're grieving. You might feel it as sorrow, melancholy, loneliness, or even despair. Physically, you might feel slowed down, heavy, or empty inside. On the other hand, joy comes from positive experiences, when we achieve something we're proud of, when we connect with others, and when we feel love and appreciation. You might feel it as happiness, elation, excitement, or just a sense of contentment. Physically, you might feel more energetic, lighter, and more open. It might seem strange, but feeling sadness can actually make our capacity for joy even deeper. When we allow ourselves to fully experience and process sadness, we create space for joy to come back into our lives. And remembering happy times can help us get through sad periods, giving us hope and making us more resilient. For example, thinking about happy memories with someone we've lost can bring up both sadness that they're gone and joy for the time we had together. This back-and-forth between sadness and joy shows us the full range of human experience and helps us appreciate how rich life is, even when things are tough. For seniors, sadness can often be connected to the loss of loved ones, changes in health or physical abilities, or shifts in social roles after retirement. It's also important to remember that joy and fulfillment are still very much possible and important in later life. Connecting with family and friends, pursuing hobbies, and reflecting on a life well-lived can bring deep satisfaction and happiness.

The Influence of Self-Talk and Thinking Habits on Sadness/Joy: Our self-talk can really affect how we experience both sadness and joy. If we tell ourselves things like "I'll never be happy again," it can make sadness last longer and feel more intense. But if we use more positive self-talk, like "It's okay to grieve, and I know I'll find joy again," it can help us get through the sadness and still appreciate the good things in our lives. In the same way, when we're feeling joyful, telling ourselves "I don't deserve this happiness" can take away from the feeling, while telling ourselves "I'm so grateful for this moment" can make it even stronger.

Emotions as Signals and Mindfulness as the Compass: Our emotions aren't just random; they're signals, giving us valuable information about what's going on inside us and how we're relating to the world around us. Fear might be telling us to be careful, anger might be a sign that someone's crossed a boundary, sadness might mean we need time to grieve and heal, and joy might be telling us that we're connecting with something important. These signals can be especially important as we age, as changes in our physical health, social connections, and life circumstances can bring about unique emotional challenges.

Mindful Response to Emotional Signals: It's important to remember that while all emotions are valid, the way we choose to express them needs to be appropriate to the situation. Instead of reacting impulsively to strong emotions, unchecked anger, for example, whether expressed through physical actions or harsh words, can damage relationships with family, friends, and others in our social circle. Mindfulness can help us become more aware of our emotional signals and choose how we respond in a healthy and constructive way, considering the potential impact of our actions and words on those around us. Mindfulness can be like having a Wise Guide or Conscious Observer inside us, helping us understand these signals without letting them control us. By practicing mindfulness, we can make better choices about how we react to our emotions instead of just reacting automatically.

Applying Mindfulness to Our Emotions: Practicing mindfulness, by focusing on our breath and bodily sensations, can help us experience these emotions fully without getting overwhelmed. Naming the emotion we are feeling—"I feel sad," or "I feel joyful"—can also help us to observe them with more clarity.

Mindfulness Exercise: Riding the Waves of Emotion

When a strong emotion arises, try this simple mindfulness exercise:

• Find a comfortable position (whether sitting or lying down) and bring your attention to your breath.

• Notice the natural rhythm of your breath as it flows in and out. As you breathe, become aware of the physical sensations associated with the emotion. Where do you feel it in your body? Is it a tightness in your chest, a knot in your stomach, or a warmth in your face?

• Simply observe these sensations without any agenda or bias, much like a surfer riding a wave. The wave rises, peaks, and eventually subsides. Similarly, you can ride the emotions that arise, intensify, and eventually pass.

• By focusing on your breath and observing the changing sensations in your body, you can ride the wave of emotion without getting swept away.

Moving Ahead with Emotional Awareness: As we've seen, our emotions aren't just isolated events; they're part of a complex, interconnected system. By understanding how emotions like fear and anger, and sadness and joy, relate to each other, we can understand our own emotional landscape much better. It can be helpful to explore other emotional pairs too, like frustration and disappointment, or excitement and anticipation. By paying attention to these connections, we can become more aware of our emotions and navigate our inner world with more skill and compassion.

Just A Little More Weighty Content To Go:

But don't worry, we are almost done with the "denser content"... In this section we weave it all together for you.

V. Embracing the Present Moment for Emotional Well-being

The Transformative Power of Now for Emotional Health: Now we finally get to merge the ideas from previous two sections that explored different aspects of "how we feel," and "what we think," and how mindfulness can play a supporting and beneficial role when working with our emotions an thoughts. Referring back, do you remember how emotions can act as signals that give us valuable information about our inner landscape, our feelings, and our relationship with the world around us? How about how we also looked at our thoughts and self-talk and thinking habits, and how they can influence our emotional signals, sometimes amplifying them, for better and worse, and sometimes even distorting their message? Well now we get to look at where mindfulness comes in as a tool to help us to both recognize and work with our inner world. First, let's take a quick look at how mindfulness, emotions, and feelings can work together.

Navigating the Complex Inner World: But how do we navigate this complex inner world more effectively? The answer is at our fingertips—it lies within our unique experience of the present moment, the only "time" we ever truly have. We can access this present moment by simply giving our awareness a gentle nudge to the "now." Using the simple tools and approaches outlined in this book, especially the gentle act of focusing on the breath, we can create some space between our emotions and our reactions giving us a buffer zone free of automatic and over-reactions.

This buffer space empowers us to investigate and reset our mental and emotional patterns and respond with greater wisdom and intention. When we're present—riding the wave of the moment—we can relax and observe our emotions without judgment or knee-jerk reactions. Instead, we can take in the whole of a situation, understand its message and relationship to us, and then choose how to respond.

Connecting Self-Awareness and Personal Growth:
Here's the key take away; by becoming more aware of our thoughts, feelings, and bodily sensations in the present moment, we are able to increasingly embody a healthy self-care approach for our personal growth, emotional well-being, leading to greater life-ease and contentment. As we learned in Section IV, Navigating the Emotional Landscape, our self-talk and related thinking and reaction habits can significantly impact our emotional experiences and perceptions.

By cultivating a gentle approach to present-moment awareness, we can start to notice these self-talk patterns—the positive and negative stories and narratives we tell ourselves—and begin to choose more helpful, supportive, less reactive inner dialogues. For example, if we are able to notice self-talk such as "I can't handle this" arising during a moment of fear or stress, we can, in time with some easy mindful tools, learn to recognize and then shift or re-frame our self-talk to something like "Wow... this is really tough, but I am sure I can manage it."

This kind of shift in our perception and ability to work with self-talk, facilitated by present-moment awareness, can significantly reduce the intensity of our fears and stress, and empower us to respond more effectively. This mindful approach can also help us better understand the underlying causes and sources of our emotional upheavals, leading to an expanded self-understanding with more effective emotional management.

Mindfulness as a Lifestyle? Maybe, Maybe Not: Don't think you have to sit around like a monk or try be mindful every waking moment to get any benefit.

And similar to other self-improvement strategies, you tend to get more benefit from your mindfulness engagement, when used with some regularity. Why? Mostly because you gain familiarity with your inner landscape which gives you some insight into how to manage any upsets. It's just like any "personal growth" tool or approach, where you choose when and how you engage with it.

We encourage you to approach mindfulness at whatever level you are comfortable and in whatever manner that resonates with you.

Mindfulness is very much an experiential tool—a valuable asset in our arsenal of life contentment, self-improvement, personal growth, a tool that can and should be tailored to your unique needs and inclinations.

Engaging Mindfulness: It doesn't take much to start experiencing the benefits of mindfulness. In Section IV, Navigating the Emotional Landscape, remember the "Riding the Wave of Emotion" exercise? The one where we used breath and body awareness to help us simply observe emotions without being overwhelmed, Do you recall how we also discussed the value of "naming our emotions" to create space and clarity? Those exercises, along with the others presented throughout the book, are all designed to help make mindfulness flexible, adaptable, accessible and beneficial. We encourage you to engage these techniques regularly (as often as you are comfortable with or drawn to). Even a small amount of regular engagement, even playful experimenting, can make a significant difference in your emotional landscape, helping to smooth out the jagged edges, allowing for a calmer and less reactive experience. And just as our fitness improves with regular participation, so too does our capacity for emotional balance, present-moment awareness, clarity, with regular gentle engagement.

Mindfulness is Not Stand-Alone Solution:

Like a nutritious meal that has all the food groups included, mindfulness, in our view, is also at its best when combined with other healthy habits, such as meaningful connections with others, healthy food choices, adequate sleep, regular physical activity, spending time in nature, and mindful consumption of media, and even getting professional support or help when needed.

End of Weighty Content!

We've covered a lot of ground in these last three sections, exploring the intricate workings of our minds and emotions. Take some time to reflect on these concepts and consider how they might apply to your own experiences. Remember, awareness is the first step toward meaningful and positive change.

VI. Looking Ahead—The Interconnectedness of Mind and Body:

In this final section and the previous one, together we've explored the groundwork for understanding how our minds work, how our thoughts and emotions intertwine, and how mindfulness can help us navigate our inner world.

Next, in Chapter 2, we'll explore the interconnectedness of mind and body, examining how our mental and emotional states directly influence our physical health and well-being, and vice versa. This understanding will provide a crucial foundation for the practical mindfulness tools and techniques we'll introduce in the following chapters, empowering you to cultivate greater emotional resilience and thrive in the face of life's inevitable ups and downs.

Chapter 2

"The body is your subconscious mind."

Candace Pert
(American Neuroscientist and Pharmacologist)

"What disturbs people's minds is not events,
but their judgments about events."

Epictetus

"The mind and body are always in conversation.
The more you listen, the better
you understand yourself."

Brenda Mapane

CHAPTER LEVEL TABLE OF CONTENTS

Chapter 2: The Interconnectedness of Mind and Body

Chapter 2

The Interconnectedness of Mind and Body

I. Introduction: Bridging Our Inner and Outer Worlds

Okay, let's review a few ideas. First, in Chapter 1, we explored several facets of mindfulness—its far-reaching implications and the subtle interplay of our thoughts and emotions. The biggest takeaway from Chapter 1 is how our thoughts, especially our thought habits and unconscious self-talk, influence our feelings—sometimes positively, sometimes not so much. We also saw how our mental state and frames of reference (life experiences) can amplify or distort the thought messages and feelings. In short, our thinking and perceptual patterns (based on our likes and dislikes) shift our perception and experience the world.

Another important concept that we introduced way back in the book's introduction and that is important to briefly reintroduce, is the idea of **"mindlessness"**—not as in an inattentive trance-like state or the loss of our identity, but rather as an open receptive awareness that is revealed once the mind and self-talk has quieted, characterized by what I refer to as **"aimlessness,"** (without self-consciousnes) a place of relaxed open awareness without effort, without agenda. The ability to simply be with our experience, without judgment or reactivity, one of the pillars of mindfulness. *(Reminder about Mindlessness from the book's introduction: This is not a goal of mindfulness per se, nor is it considered something that is "better" than other ways of experiencing the present moment. It's simply another aspect or experience potential that may naturally arise as part of the rich landscape of mindful engagement.)*

Now, let's turn our attention to a crucial element: the profound connection between our minds and our bodies—our physical and emotional health, our physical and emotional well-being. We'll explore this connection from both philosophical and scientific perspectives (I promise, just enough of each to showcase the transformative potential of mindfulness). This "mindfulness bridge" we're building will connect these ideas to the foundational principles of how we live, interact with others, and move through the world.

By exploring the whole of the mind/body/emotions/feelings synergy, we'll start to see how each element affects the others, directly affecting our physical and mental health, as well as our overall well-being. This intricate interplay is especially relevant as we age, affording opportunities to influence our physical health, mood, thinking, cognitive abilities, and overall well-being and emotional resilience, helping us shift out of any negative patterns we may have developed.

Ancient Wisdom, Modern Science

The mind-body connection is a cornerstone of both traditional spiritual wisdom and contemporary scientific understanding. Mindfulness offers a holistic approach to well-being, benefiting both mental and physical health and touched upon in this chapter.

II. The Body's Silent Language

Everyday Examples of the Mind-Body Connection

What do butterflies in your stomach, a clenched jaw, and tense shoulders have in common? They all illustrate the mind-body connection. Most of us have experienced butterflies before a presentation, a clenched jaw when angry or resolute, or tension headaches and shoulder aches after a stressful day (or even a visit to the dentist). These everyday examples show how our thoughts, emotions, and feelings can manifest as physical sensations. While these fleeting symptoms might seem like a normal part of life, this connection goes much further, influencing our physical discomforts or shaping our shape our posture, facial expressions, then can even impact bodily functions— affecting everything from our mood and thought patterns to our overall sense of well-being and outlook on life. Our bodies constantly send us signals, both subtle and obvious, that are not only a reflection of our inner state, but a valuable tool to keeping tabs on our health and overall well- being.

Beyond Mindfulness: When to Seek Medical Care

It's important to understand that at the more extreme end of the mind-body connection spectrum, there can be far more serious physical signals that go beyond the ability of mindfulness to address. Always seek appropriate and timely medical care, including emergency care, when needed.

The Mind-Body Connection and Aging

For seniors, the mind-body connection can be particularly pronounced. As we age, we may experience more aches and pains, raising the question: "What came first—the problem or the pain?" This "chicken-and-egg" scenario can make it difficult to determine whether a discomfort is a medical issue, a habitual stress response, or simply tension from chronic pain of a challenging interaction or unexpected bad news. As our bodies change with age, we need to become "mindful sleuths"—body-mind detectives—not only becoming aware of physical changes and their associated discomforts or limitations but also understanding whether those discomforts are:

- Related to external stressors,

- Related to mental or emotional patterns, or

- A sign of a medical condition requiring a doctor's visit.

Regardless of the source, these discomforts can significantly impact our emotional and mental well-being. For example:

- Chronic pain can lead to frustration, irritability, or even depression.

- Changes in mobility or energy levels can affect our sense of independence and self-esteem.

Conversely, engaging in enjoyable activities, like spending time with loved, pursuing hobbies, or spending time in nature, can boost our mood and energy, demonstrating the positive feedback loop between mind and body.

Recognizing the Signals (Good and Bad)

Let's see if we can make this more tangible. Take a moment to relax while you're reading this book. Close your eyes and recall a time when you were worried, anxious, or tense about a health issue. Do you remember any physical symptoms, such as:

- A racing pulse

- Digestive problems, or

- Difficulty sleeping?

These experiences illustrate how worries and anxieties can directly affect the body. Now, try the opposite: recall a time of joy, contentment, or gratitude. Do you notice a different set of physical sensations—perhaps:

- A lighter mood,

- Increased energy, or

- A sense of ease?

These examples demonstrate the power of the mind-body connection and hopefully, show why we are starting to explore this important mind/body relationship.

Connecting to Present Moment Awareness

These subjective experiences—physical pain, tension, and emotional tension (worry, anxiety, catastrophizing)—are not random; they reflect the constant communication between mind and body. Through the process of beginning to cultivate present-moment awareness (as discussed in Chapter 1), we can become more attuned to these signals, both subtle and the more obvious ones. By becoming familiar with and exploring our present-moment awareness capacity, we can learn to recognize our early signs of stress, anxiety, or other emotional states before they escalate and derail our sense of well-being and ease. This empowers us to respond proactively rather than reactively, using the mindfulness tools we'll explore in later chapters to help us cultivate active self-care patterns by attuning our awareness to be sensitive to our emotional, thought-based, or physical discomforts.

III. Scientific & Spiritual Perspectives on the Mind-Body Connection

The profound connection between mind and body has been explored for centuries, both through the lens of scientific inquiry and the wisdom of ancient and contemporary spiritual traditions. This section examines this two perspectives, drawing upon research from various scientific disciplines to illuminate the impact of our thoughts, emotions, and experiences on our physical health. Alongside these scientific findings, we'll also explore the perspectives of spiritual traditions, which have long emphasized the importance of cultivating inner peace and well-being for overall health and harmony. My goal is to provide you with important insights into the profound connection between our minds and bodies, drawing upon both contemporary scientific understanding and time-honored spiritual perspectives and practices. Let's dive in...

Weighty Content Ahead:

Take it easy with this next science-heavy section. There is a lot to absorb and consider.

Neurology (The Nervous System & Neuroplasticity):

The nervous system serves as the body's primary communication network, acting as a complex two-way system. It not only facilitates the transmission of signals from the brain to every part of the body—organs, muscles, glands, and other systems—managing their function, but it also receives and processes sensory information from the body and the environment (such as pain, light, and temperature), providing a constant stream of feedback to the brain. This remarkable system is also capable of change and adaptation throughout our lives, a phenomenon known as neuroplasticity.

Neuroplasticity refers to the brain's ability to reorganize itself by forming new neural connections. Think of your brain as a garden. Mindfulness can help you create new pathways and strengthen the ones you use most, especially those associated with attention, emotional regulation, and self-awareness. Research suggests that mindfulness practices can induce both structural and functional changes in the brain, supporting this process of neuroplasticity.

Neuroplasticity: The Brain's Adaptability

Neuroplasticity is the brain's ability to change and adapt throughout life. It's not just for kids! Our brains are constantly rewiring themselves based on our experiences, thoughts, and actions. Mindfulness, by focusing attention and cultivating awareness, can influence this process, strengthening neural pathways associated with positive mental and emotional states. This is why mindfulness can be so effective in promoting well-being at any age.

Neurology & Spiritual Perspectives: Cultivating Awareness and Inner Transformation

Many spiritual traditions emphasize the cultivation of focused attention and awareness as a means of achieving inner peace and transformative shifts in consciousness. These practices, such as meditation, contemplative prayer, mindfulness, and yoga, can be understood as intentional exercises in neuroplasticity, strengthening neural pathways associated with positive mental and emotional states.

From a spiritual perspective, the nervous system can be seen as the physical embodiment of our consciousness, and by intentionally shaping our thoughts and attention, we can influence the very structure and function of our brains.

These practices are not just about feeling good; they can lead to profound changes in how we perceive ourselves and the world around us, fostering greater self-awareness, compassion, and wisdom. For example, some contemplative traditions believe that consistent meditation practice can lead to the development of specific qualities like equanimity and loving-kindness, which are reflected in the neural circuitry of the brain. By engaging in these practices, we are not only tending to our mental and emotional well-being but also actively participating in our own spiritual growth and transformation.

Cardiology (The Stress Response & Impact on Cardiovascular Health):

As you likely know, cardiologists focus on the heart and circulatory system. Studies in this field have shown how stress activates the body's "fight-or-flight" response, triggering the release of hormones like cortisol (a steroid hormone produced by the adrenal glands). While this response is helpful in short bursts, chronic stress—resulting in long-term elevated levels of cortisol—can negatively impact cardiovascular health, increasing the risk of heart disease and contributing to elevated or long-term high blood pressure.

Mindfulness engagement has been shown to help regulate the stress response by reducing cortisol levels, leading to lower blood pressure and supporting healthier heart function.

Cardiology & Spiritual Perspectives: Spiritual Practices for Stress Regulation and Heart Health

Many spiritual traditions recognize the profound connection between our mental and emotional state and our physical well-being, particularly the health of the cardiovascular system. The concept of regulating the stress response through various approaches is central to these traditions, which emphasize the importance of cultivating inner peace and tranquility for overall well-being. Techniques such as breath-work, meditation, mindfulness, yoga, and Tai Chi are often used to calm the nervous system, reduce stress hormones like cortisol, and promote a sense of inner balance.

These approaches are not just about feeling good; they can have a tangible impact on heart health by lowering blood pressure, improving circulation, and reducing the risk of heart disease. For example, studies have shown that regular meditation can be as effective as medication in lowering blood pressure in some individuals. By integrating these spiritual techniques into our lives, we can support not only our mental and emotional well-being but also the health of our hearts.

Psychology (Impact of Emotions on the Body & Benefits of Mindfulness for Mental Health):

Psychologists study the mind and behavior, exploring the powerful link between emotions and physical health. Research demonstrates how chronic stress and negative emotions can contribute to various health issues, including anxiety, depression, and weakened immune function. Studies also show the benefits of mindfulness for effectively managing stress, improving mood, and enhancing overall mental well-being.

Psychology & Spiritual Perspectives: Emotional Balance, Resilience, and Inner Strength

Spiritual traditions have long recognized the powerful influence of our emotions on our overall well-being.

Many offer practices, such as meditation, contemplation, mindfulness, and self-inquiry, that are designed to help individuals understand and manage their emotions, fostering greater emotional balance and resilience. These practices often emphasize the importance of self-awareness and acceptance as key components of emotional healing and growth.

From a spiritual perspective, our emotions are not something to be suppressed or avoided, but rather valuable sources of information about our inner world. By taking a mindful approach, we are allowing our disruptive emotions to recede which allows our inherent compassion to be revealed. By gently observing our emotions without any agenda or bias, we can begin to see and understand their underlying causes, and naturally respond to them with greater calm, grace, and ease.

This process can lead to balanced emotional regulation, reduced reactivity, and a greater sense of contentment and well-being. For example, some contemplative traditions teach that by simply observing our emotions with neutral awareness, the grip of emotional upheaval is loosened, and a relaxed natural freedom from the cycles of reactivity, anxiety, and suffering is revealed.

Pain Management (The Role of the Mind in Pain Perception):

Specialists in pain management understand that pain is not solely a physical sensation; it is also significantly influenced by psychological, emotional, and cognitive factors. Mindfulness techniques, as used in pain management, can help individuals manage chronic pain by shifting their relationship to sensations and experience of pain.

Rather than struggling against or being overwhelmed by the pain, mindfulness encourages a relaxed and open observation of the present moment experience, including the pain itself *(See Chapter 8: Mindfulness for Pain & Discomfort)*. This shift in perspective and approach to "meeting pain" can reduce the suffering and anxiety associated with pain which is supportive of improved quality of life. Mindfulness is often used as part of a comprehensive pain management plan that may also include medication, physical therapy, and other interventions.

Pain Management & Spiritual Perspectives: Transcending Pain and Cultivating Inner Calm

Many spiritual traditions address the nature of suffering and offer practices for coping with physical and emotional pain. Concepts like acceptance, non-attachment, and finding meaning in suffering are often explored as ways to transcend physical discomfort and find inner peace.

From a spiritual perspective, pain is not just a physical sensation; it's also a complex experience shaped by our thoughts, emotions, and beliefs. Mindfulness techniques, such as mindful breathing, body scan/body awareness exercises, and various kindness visualizations, can help us shift our relationship to pain sensations.

Geriatric Medicine (Mind-Body Connection and Aging):

Geriatric medicine focuses on the healthcare of older adults, recognizing the unique challenges that accompany aging. Research in this field highlights the importance of the mind-body connection for maintaining physical and cognitive function in seniors. Mindfulness practices have been shown to improve sleep, reduce stress, and enhance cognitive function in older adults.

Geriatric Medicine & Spiritual Perspectives: Finding Meaning and Purpose in Aging

Many spiritual traditions offer practices and teachings that support healthy aging, emphasizing the importance of maintaining mental clarity, emotional balance, and a sense of purpose throughout life. Techniques such as meditation, yoga, tai chi, mindfulness, and contemplative prayer are often recommended to promote physical and mental well-being in seniors.

From a spiritual perspective, aging is not just a process of decline, but also an opportunity for growth, wisdom, and deeper connection with ourselves and the world around us. As we age, our priorities may shift, and we may have more time for reflection and introspection.

Spiritual approaches can help us navigate these transitions with calm, grace, and emotional resilience, allowing us to explore meaning and purpose in these new chapters of life. Additionally, these same approaches can also help us to recognize and embrace a sense of gratitude for the experiences we've had, accept the changes that come with aging, and meet the present moment with greater appreciation.

By connecting with our inner selves and cultivating a sense of connection to something larger than ourselves, we can enjoy a fulfilling sense of contentment, and relax into a greater sense fulfillment for the later stages of life.

Other Research (Including DNA Research and Mindfulness):

Beyond the specific fields discussed, other research areas are also exploring the mind-body connection at a deeper level. For example, research on gene expression—how our genes are read and acted upon by our cells—suggests that our experiences, including our mental and emotional states, can influence which genes are turned "on" or "off."

Think of our genes as a set of instructions, and gene expression as how those instructions are followed.

Just like a conductor can choose which instruments play in an orchestra, our experiences can influence which genes are expressed, impacting our health and sense of well-being. Mindfulness techniques can help us embody positive mental states, which can play a role in supporting the expression of genes linked to well-being and health.

Conversely, upsetting or agitated mental states, such as chronic stress, have the potential to affect the expression of genes associated with inflammation or other detrimental health effects.

Gene Expression and Mindfulness

Gene expression is a dynamic process, constantly changing in response to our internal and external environment. It's not just about the genes we inherit; it's about how those genes are expressed – how they're activated or silenced. Mindfulness, by influencing our mental and emotional states, can potentially affect this process. Research suggests that mindfulness practices may help regulate gene expression in ways that promote health and well-being, potentially by reducing the expression of genes linked to inflammation and stress. This highlights the profound interconnectedness of mind and body, showing how our thoughts and feelings can influence our biology at a cellular level.

Other Research & Spiritual Perspectives: The Interconnectedness of Mind, Body, and Spirit

Many spiritual traditions have long emphasized the transformative power of inner work and the ability of the mind to influence the body. These insights, now being explored through scientific research like studies on gene expression, further highlight the importance of cultivating inner peace and well-being.

From a spiritual perspective, our thoughts, emotions, and experiences not only affect our physical health but also our spiritual well-being.

The concept of interconnectedness is central to many spiritual teachings, suggesting that we are all part of a larger web of life and that our actions and intentions have ripple effects throughout this web.

Mindfulness strategies that support positive mental states, may, according to preliminary research, play a role in influencing gene expression in ways could be beneficial. Conversely, negative mental states, such as chronic stress, may potentially influence gene expression in ways that are less beneficial.

While further research is needed to fully understand these complex interactions, these practices are not just about individual well-being; they're about recognizing our interconnectedness with all beings and cultivating a sense of responsibility for the well-being of the whole. By tending to our inner landscape, we are not only healing ourselves but also contributing to the healing of the world around us.

End of Weighty Content:

Time to relax and get ready for some "easy and enjoyable" mindfulness exercises in the upcoming Chapter 3.

IV. Concluding Thoughts on the Mind-Body Connection:

This section has presented a more in-depth exploration of the remarkable interplay between mind and body, drawing upon both the rigorous findings of scientific research and the timeless wisdom of spiritual traditions.

We've seen how several scientific disciplines, from neurology to cardiology and beyond, offer compelling evidence for the powerful influence of our thoughts, emotions, and experiences on our physical health. From regulating the stress response to potentially influencing gene expression, science increasingly validates the ancient understanding of the mind-body connection.

Furthermore, together we've explored how diverse spiritual traditions offer a rich tapestry of practices and perspectives that complement and deepen our understanding of this connection. These traditions emphasize not only the importance of mental and emotional well-being, but also the interconnectedness of mind, body, and spirit, offering pathways to cultivate inner peace, resilience, and a sense of meaning and purpose. This integrated understanding empowers us to take proactive steps to enhance our overall well-being, including our physical, emotional, and spiritual dimensions.

V. Getting Ready for Chapter 3 Where We Start to Experience Our Body-Mind Connection Through Mindfulness:

Now that we've completed our overview of the scientific and spiritual perspectives on the mind-body connection, in the next chapter we move forward with a few very simple mindfulness exercises designed to help you experience the mind-body connection directly.

About An Easy Mindful Moments Approach: We'll begin with a series of what I like to call "mindful moment" exercises—very simple exercises that can be easily adapted and integrated into any situation (indoors, outdoors, active, or at rest).

Whether you find yourself in a challenging circumstance (emotional, physical, or mental) or simply in the midst of a pleasurable moment, these mindful moment exercises are tailor-made for both beginners and those more familiar with mindfulness techniques.

The beauty of these exercises is that they require only a moment of your time and your willingness to briefly and gently refocus your attention. And remember, no matter what level of focus you bring to the exercise, that is the perfect level for YOU! The key is to approach these exercises with gentle curiosity and without any pressure to achieve a particular outcome. Simply notice what arises, allowing yourself to be present with your experience.

Big Rewards in a Small Package: Despite the outwardly simple appearance of our mindful moment exercises, they are potent tools that can support any level mindfulness engagement you undertake—whether formalized or on-demand and as needed—they are surprisingly effective and restorative.

Not only can they serve as a foundation for deeper mindfulness explorations, but they can also act as a perfect "quick reset" when you find your mind or emotions out of balance.

Think of the "mindful moments" as a small ball of malleable clay—simple yet capable of being shaped and molded into countless forms to help you meet life head-on. Adaptable to a wide range of abilities and needs, they are an easy-to-add, fast-to-do, and scalable option for your daily routine.

Chapter 3

"Every moment is a fresh beginning."

T.S. Eliot

"In the beginner's mind
there are many possibilities,
but in the expert's there are few."

Shunryu Suzuki

"The moment one gives close attention
to anything, even a blade of grass,
it becomes a mysterious, awesome,
indescribably magnificent world in itself."

Henry Miller

CHAPTER LEVEL TABLE OF CONTENTS

Chapter 3: Mindful Moment Explorations

Chapter 3

Mindful Moment Explorations

I. A Simple Approach to Mindfulness:
Easy, Adaptable, and Flexible Exercises

The techniques I outline in this chapter introduce the foundational elements of mindfulness. Most of what follows in this chapter focuses on bringing awareness to a single sensation or action—these are what we call "mindful moments," like focusing on a single breath or the feeling of one object in your hand. Others involve gently exploring sensations within a specific part of your body, as in the last exercise in this chapter, the "One Hand."

These approaches are designed to be accessible to everyone, regardless of prior experience with mindfulness or physical ability or lack thereof. You can think of these exercises as building blocks—simple in their individual form, yet flexible in their ability to be extended, expanded, and combined to create longer and more in-depth mindfulness experiences, some of which we will explore in later chapters.

As you may know, there are many different approaches to mindfulness, ranging from these sorts of brief exercises to far more elaborate techniques cultivated over a lifetime. My focus here is to provide a solid grounding in these fundamental practices so you can easily and directly experience the mind-body connection and use them as helpful tools in your own life.

The Story Behind These Mindful Moments: My own introduction to the power of these mindful moments came during a challenging session with my therapist at a time in my life when I was facing a variety of personal challenges. The therapist I was working with also happened to be an Aikido instructor and was well-versed in his students' practices, their mental blocks, and their own perceived shortcomings. During one exchange I was lamenting that my own meditation practice sessions were "not long enough" or "not performed well enough" or some other similar sentiment. After I had finished expressing my concerns, he paused and then asked me one question:

"What about taking one breath with full awareness... Would that be enough?" He wasn't suggesting some unattainable ideal, but simply bringing my full attention, at whatever level I was able to apply, to that single breath, just as it was.

That one profound exchange forever changed my perspective on mindfulness and meditation... And freed me from the burden of worrying about whether my efforts were "long enough," releasing me from the trap of "shoulds," and allowing me to set aside the pursuit of a "perfect outcome or approach."

It is from that insightful exchange, combined with my sincere desire to make the benefits of mindfulness easily accessible and enjoyable, that we offer these gentle exercises and tools.

But What About?: Before we get to the exercises, let's address a couple of common concerns many people have about mindfulness. These are:

- That it will make them less productive

- That it requires a significant time commitment

- That they can't dedicate their whole day to being mindful

If you share these concerns, you're in good company. Many people find themselves thinking, "I don't have time for mindfulness," or "Everything takes too long when I try to do it mindfully!," or "I am too busy for mindfulness."

In our busy, get-things-done society, the idea of "being mindful" can indeed seem like mindfulness is the opposite of "getting things done" and that it is just a slow-moving, unproductive activity—even maybe even a bit foreign or woo-woo. We're often told that "doing more" equates to a "better life," and "not being busy" is often equated with being lazy (or worse).

But what if we told you that mindfulness could be adapted to fit into your life easily, requiring only a few moments as-needed or when-wanted?

What if, instead of being another item on your to-do list, mindfulness became a tool to not only ease life's challenges and make our upsets a little less...flammable, but also enhance our ability to savor life?

My approach and philosophy for mindfulness is gentle and simple: Share easy-to-use tools and exercises that can help you discover and create a life where you begin to release the shackles of a lifetime of unchallenged assumptions, stuck mental routines, and reactive emotional patterns. A personal "reset" button if you will, a gentler and more receptive life view—like the push of fresh air rushing in through a newly opened window, allowing us to experience life more fully, connect more deeply with ourselves and others, and appreciate the profound interconnectedness of our minds and bodies and our amazing relationship with the world around us.

The following easy exercises offer practical ways to cultivate this gentle and expanded awareness in your day-to-day life.

II. Five Mindful Moment Exercises

Now that we've explored the foundational ideas of mindfulness, let's put them into action with these "Mindful Moment Exercises." They're designed to be brief, easy, and safe, offering a simple way to gently engage a mindful approach to connect with your thoughts, emotions, and body, no matter your level of experience, interest level, or current circumstances.

Mindful Moment One: One Breath

We're starting with what I simply call the "One Breath"— perhaps the easiest of all mindfulness exercises. I think of it as a gateway, or even a launchpad, to all mindfulness explorations, whether those presented here in this book, or any others you may encounter.

This simple yet effective foundational exercise is a fantastic tool you can use anytime, anywhere. Feeling a surge of anger or frustration? You might try taking a breath. Feeling a bit of pain or physical discomfort? You might try taking a breath. Feeling overwhelmed with worry? Taking a breath can help. Even enjoying a pleasant moment? Take a breath!

I invite you to simply take one mindful breath.

This one-breath technique is like taking one step forward in the direction you want to go. It helps reset your current experience—especially challenging ones—by gently shifting your focus from the challenge, pain, situation, frustration, etc., to a wider, more relaxed perspective. It invites you to move from a reactive or overwhelmed state to a place where you can begin to choose another reaction or a different course of action.

The simple act of focusing on a single breath can be a wonderful part of your day, helping you navigate difficult moments or simply relax and savor the good ones. It's a quick and easy way to reduce stress, gently settle into a wider awareness, shift perspectives, and even enhance your enjoyment of life.

The Exercise: An Invitation to Explore

First, I invite you to rest in a comfortable position. Sitting, standing, leaning against a wall, or even lying down are all OK. **You might choose to gently close your eyes.** (Closing your eyes is optional, but closing your eyes can help you focus inward, but it's perfectly fine to keep them open if you prefer.)

• **You are invited to take one slow, conscious breath.** At your own pace, following the inhalation all the way through to the end of the exhalation.

• **Notice the sensations.** Notice the sensation of the air as it enters and leaves your body—the air in your mouth or nostrils, the rise and fall of your chest or abdomen, feelings of relaxation or tension, etc.

- **Gently return to your activity.** Once your breath is finished, gently open your eyes (if closed) and simply return your awareness to your current activity.

Modifications for Limited Mobility:

Comfort and ease are key. If sitting or standing is uncomfortable, you can perform this practice while lying down. If lying down is uncomfortable, try a reclined position, either in a chair or with head elevation on a bed. Using a walker or other supportive device? Simply rest in the support of your device (walker, crutches, cane, wheelchair). If focusing on the breath is difficult, you could focus on another sensation, such as the feeling of your feet on the floor or your hands in your lap, or even the feel of the air on your cheeks.

Gently Expanding the Practice:

If you're so inclined, there are two ways to gently expand this practice. The first is to simply repeat the one-breath cycle. This approach can be particularly helpful if you find that a single breath hasn't brought sufficient calm in a challenging situation. The second approach is to set the intention before you begin, to take several breaths instead of just one. For example, you might decide to take three mindful breaths or five or more. No matter which approach you choose, the important point is to go at your own pace.

More breaths are not "better"—it's far more valuable to be fully present with a single breath than to decide "I will do three!," and then lose focus after the first. *Baby steps and small "wins" are our friends!*

Mindful Moment Two: One Thing

Now, let's explore the familiar world around you by putting your attention on just one simple, everyday object. I think you will find that through a subtle shift in our patterns of observation, even the most ordinary things can reveal a world of wonder right at our fingertips, leading us to an expanded appreciation of the normally taken-for-granted things around us. Think of the One-Thing exercise as a playful exploration, a chance to discover and rediscover the simple joys of connecting deeply with your senses.

The Exercise: An Invitation to Explore

First, choose your object: You are invited to find a small, easily held object. A pebble or small stone works well, offering a variety of textures and visual details, but you could also use a piece of fruit (like an apple or orange), a utensil (like a spoon or fork), a leaf, or any other small, safe object you have on hand. Choose something that feels comfortable to hold and that you can easily observe.

• **Holding the object:** You are invited to gently cradle the object in your palm. Notice its weight and heft. How does it feel in your palm? Is it light or heavy? Can you find its balance point using one finger? You might explore how the weight shifts as you move your hand slightly or how the balance changes as you reposition your object.

• **Exploring its texture:** You are invited to run your fingers over the surface. Is it smooth, rough, bumpy, or a combination of textures? Notice any irregularities, damage, blemishes, or sharp edges. Pay attention to the subtle sensations in your fingertips as they interact with the object's surface.

• **Observing its appearance:** Look closely at the object. What color or colors do you see? What shape is it? Are there any patterns or markings? Notice the details you might not normally see—the subtle variations in color, the way light reflects off its surface, the tiny lines and crevices.

• **(Optional) Exploring the sound:** If applicable (like with a pebble or utensil), you might gently tap the object on a surface or scratch it with a fingernail. What sound does it make? Is it a sharp tap, a dull thud, or a soft scraping sound? Notice the quality of the sound and how it resonates.

• *Playing with your exploration:* You might try holding the object in different ways—in your other hand, up to the light, upside down. See how it naturally rests on a flat surface.

(Exercise continues next page)

• **Explore it from different angles & perspectives:** Notice how these different perspectives change your experience of the object.

• **Bringing your full attention to the object:** For a few moments, you are invited to simply be present with the object, noticing all the sensations it evokes. Allow yourself to be fully absorbed in the experience, gently allowing thoughts or distractions simply arise and fall away.

• **Gently releasing the object:** When you're ready, you are invited to gently set the object down and return your attention to your surroundings. Take a moment to notice how you feel after this brief exploration. With a mindful breath or two, gently return to your attention back to your surroundings.

Modifications for Limited Mobility:

Comfort and ease are key. If holding the object in your hand is difficult, you can place it on a stable surface in front of you and explore it visually. If touching the object is challenging, focus on the visual aspects, noticing its color, shape, and details. If focusing on the object is difficult, you may choose to focus on a sensation in your body such as the feeling of your feet on the ground or the feeling of your breath moving in and out of your body.

Gently Expanding the Practice:

If you're so inclined, there are two ways to gently expand this practice. The first is to simply repeat or extend the time you take exploring the same object, noticing if your experience changes with repeated or extended observation. This approach can be particularly helpful if you find your mind wandering or if you want to deepen your connection or experience with the object. The second approach is to choose a new object and repeat the exercise. For example, you might explore a pebble and then a leaf, noticing the differences in your experience. No matter which approach you choose, the important point is to go at your own pace. More explorations are not "better"—it's far more valuable to be fully present with a single object than to rush through multiple objects without full attention. Baby steps and small "wins" are our friends!

Mindful Moment Three: One Taste

Let's explore the simple act of tasting by focusing all your attention on just one bite of food. Think of it as a chance to rekindle your relationship with flavor, to rediscover the amazing richness of sensory experience and cultivate a deeper appreciation for the present moment. By bringing mindful attention to that single bite, you can rediscover the amazing richness of sensory experience and cultivate a deeper appreciation for the present moment. Instead of focusing on hunger, we're focusing on savoring every sensation associated with that one bite.

The Exercise: An Invitation to Explore

First, choose your bite: You are invited to select a small amount of food that you enjoy and that is safe for you to eat, considering any dietary restrictions or allergies you may have. Here are some options you might consider:

- A bite of a simple sandwich (like a cheese sandwich)

- One spoonful of cottage cheese or applesauce

- A small piece of plain or buttered toast

- A tasty piece of a favorite vegetable (cooked or raw)

- One sip of tea or broth

- One bite of your favorite fruit

- A small bite of a cracker or cookie

Now, with your chosen "bite" you can begin:

- **Observe the food:** Before taking a bite, you are invited to take a moment to look at the food. Notice its color(s), shape, and texture. Is it wet, shiny, smooth, or rough? You might allow yourself to anticipate the taste and texture.

• **Smell the food:** You might bring the food closer to your nose and gently inhale. Notice any aromas or scents. What do you smell?

• **Hold the food:** If appropriate, you might hold the food in your hand or between your fingers before bringing it to your mouth. Notice the texture against your fingers.

• **Take just one bite/sip:** You are invited to bring the food to your mouth and take just one small bite or sip.

• **Experiencing the texture:** Notice the texture of the food as it touches or passes your lips and then your tongue. What does it feel like?

• **Tasting the food:** You might allow the food to rest in your mouth or cheek or on your tongue for a moment before you begin to chew. Notice the initial flavors that arise and the flavors that follow.

• **Chewing slowly and mindfully:** If the food requires chewing, you are invited to chew slowly and mindfully, paying attention to the sensations in your mouth—the texture as you chew, the pressure on your teeth, the movement of your jaw, the mixing of the food with your saliva. Notice how the flavors change as you chew.

• **Swallowing mindfully:** When you're ready, you are invited to swallow the food, noticing the sensation of it moving down your throat.

(Exercise continues next page)

• **Noticing the aftertaste:** After you've swallowed, you might take a moment to notice any lingering flavors or sensations in your mouth.

• **Noticing any emotions:** As you experience the taste, notice any emotions that arise. Do you feel satisfaction, contentment, gratitude, or joy? Do you notice any anticipation or salivation before you take the bite? You are invited to simply observe these emotions without judgment.

• **Returning to your surroundings:** Once the experience of the one bite is complete, you are invited to gently return your attention to your surroundings.

Modifications for Limited Mobility:

Comfort and ease are key. If holding food in your hand or bringing it to your mouth is difficult, you can have a caregiver or helper assist you. You can also place the food on a stable surface in front of you and focus on enjoying the scent and the way the food looks. If chewing or swallowing is challenging, choose a food with a softer texture, such as applesauce or broth. If focusing on the food is difficult, you could choose to focus on a sensation in your body such as the feeling of your feet on the ground or the feeling of your breath moving in and out of your body.

Gently Expanding the Practice:

If you're so inclined, there are two ways to gently expand this practice. The first is to simply repeat the exploration with another bite, noticing if your experience changes with repeated tasting. This approach can be particularly helpful if you find your mind wandering or if you want to deepen your connection with the flavor. The second approach is to choose a new bite of a different food and repeat the exercise. For example, you might explore a bite of apple and then a bite of cheese, noticing the differences in your experience. No matter which approach you choose, the important point is to go at your own pace. More explorations are not "better"—it's far more valuable to be fully present with a single bite than to rush through multiple bites without full attention. Remember, baby steps and small "wins" are our friends!

Mindful Moment Four: Your Soundscape

Let's explore the often-unnoticed symphony of sound all around you. By bringing a mindful appreciation to the sounds you encounter, you can reveal a deeper connection to the present moment, unveiling a complex soundscape that often goes unheard, simply by refocusing your sense of hearing. Instead of listening for something specific, we're simply suggesting to opening our ears and minds to all the varied and rich sounds that are already there, just waiting to be discovered and enjoyed right now.

(Exercise continues next page)

The Exercise: An Invitation to Explore

First, you are invited to find a comfortable position.
You can practice this exercise indoors or outdoors, wherever
you feel at ease.

- **Become aware of the soundscape:** Simply become
aware of the sounds around you. There's no need to focus
on any one sound in particular. Simply allow the sounds
to come and go in your awareness.

- **Gently close your eyes (optional):** Closing your
eyes can help you focus more fully on what you are
hearing by minimizing the often overpowering visual
sense. If you prefer to keep your eyes open, try a soft,
unfocused gaze. This means allowing your eyes to rest
gently on a single point or area without focusing on any
specific details.

- **Notice the qualities of sound:** As you listen, you are
invited to notice the different qualities of the sounds you
hear. Are they loud or soft? High-pitched or low-pitched?
Close by or far away? Do they have a distinct rhythm or
pattern?

- **Acknowledge all sounds:** Notice all the sounds that
arise, whether they are pleasant or unpleasant, expected
or unexpected. You might hear natural sounds like
birdsong or wind, household sounds like the ticking of
a clock or the hum of a refrigerator, human sounds like

conversations or laughter, the rustling of your clothing, or even internal sounds like your heartbeat or stomach gurgling. You are invited to simply acknowledge each sound without bias or agenda.

• **Working with hearing challenges:** If you experience hearing loss or tinnitus (ringing in the ears), you are invited to simply focus on the sounds you can hear, even if they are faint or muffled. If tinnitus is present, you are invited to simply include it as part of the soundscape you are observing.

• **Maintain a receptive attitude:** As you listen, simply relax into what you are hearing. There's no need to try to block out any sounds or label them as "good" or "bad." You are invited to simply observe the experience of hearing itself. And if that little voice inside starts to give a running commentary on what you are hearing, just let that voice fade away just as the sounds also fade away.

• **Connect to daily life:** Throughout your day, you might try bringing this mindful awareness to sound into your daily activities. Notice the sounds as you move through your home, walk in your neighborhood, sit at your desk, or engage in conversations with others.

• **Gently conclude the practice:** When you're ready, you are invited to gently open your eyes (if closed) and with a mindful breath or two, return your attention to your surroundings.

Modifications for Limited Mobility:

Comfort and ease are key. You can practice this exercise in any comfortable position, whether sitting, lying down, or reclining. If changing positions is difficult, simply remain in your current position and bring your awareness to the sounds around you. If focusing on external sounds is challenging, you could focus on internal sounds, such as your heartbeat or the sound of your breath.

Gently Expanding the Practice:

If you're so inclined, there are a couple of ways to gently expand this practice. The first is to focus your attention on a single sound for a longer period, noticing how its qualities change over time. For example, you might focus on the sounds of the city and their changes over time, or the call-and-response of birdsong. The second approach is to intentionally shift your attention from one sound to another, noticing how your awareness moves and shifts. No matter which approach you choose, the important point is to go at your own pace. More explorations are not "better"— it's far more valuable to be fully present with a single sound than to rush through multiple sounds without full attention. Again, baby steps and small "wins" are our friends!

Mindful Moment Five: One Hand

Now it's time to add a little depth to our explorations in an experiential look at "One Hand". Just think about it: Our hands are constantly busy doing stuff, interacting with the world in countless ways, yet how often do we truly notice them or appreciate them? By taking a few moments for a mindful exploration of one hand—noticing sensations, movement, appearance, and areas of discomfort or limitation—you can start the journey to a richer appreciation of your body's forms and functions, while also deepening your awareness and connection to a world so often passed by.

The Exercise: An Invitation to Explore:

First, you are invited to find a comfortable position. You might sit or lie down in a position that allows you to comfortably observe and explore one of your hands. You can rest your hand on your lap, on a table, or hold it gently in your other hand.

• **Beginning at the wrist:** You are invited to bring your attention to your wrist. Notice any sensations present— warmth, coolness, tingling, or simply the feeling of your wrist against your clothing or the surface it's resting on. If you choose you can also explore your wrist with your other hand, gently tracing the contours of your wrist.

(Exercise continues next page)

• **Exploring the hand, moving outward:** You are invited to gently move your attention from your wrist down through the rest of your hand. Notice the back of your hand, your palm, and the edges of your hand. Again, if you choose you can also explore these areas with your other hand, gently tracing them.

• **Paying attention to the hand movements:** As you shift your awareness, begin to explore places where your hand moves—your knuckles, the joints in your fingers, and your wrist. Once more, if you are so inclined, use your free hand to also gentle trace the contours of your joints while you are moving your hand.

• **Exploring the fingers:** Now you are invited to bring your attention to your fingers. You can explore all of your fingers at once, noticing the overall sensation, or you can explore each finger individually, moving your attention from one fingertip to the next. Again, using your free hand to trace the contours of your fingers if you are so inclined.

• **Noticing physical sensations:** As you move your attention through your hand, you are invited to notice all physical sensations that arise. Do you feel any warmth, coolness, tingling, pressure, or subtle vibrations?

• **Exploring range of motion and flexibility:** You might gently wiggle your fingers and rotate your wrist. Notice the range of motion and any feelings of flexibility or stiffness.

• **Noticing any pain or discomfort:** If you experience any pain or discomfort in your hand, you are invited to simply acknowledge it without judgment. Notice the location of the pain (knuckle, finger, wrist, etc.) and the type of pain (sharp, dull, aching, shooting). Notice if the pain changes with movement or rest. (And please don't do anything that aggravates any pain or discomfort you are feeling)

• **Observing the appearance of your hand:** You might take a moment to look at your hand. Notice its color(s), the visual texture of the skin, and whether it appears dry or moist. Try looking at your hand from different angles, perhaps even back-lighting it with a lamp or window, noticing its translucent quality.

• **Exploring the feeling of touch:** Apart from tracing the hand's contours mentioned above, you might gently hold your hand with your other hand. Notice the sensations of contact, warmth, and pressure. If you have someone with you, you may consider asking them to gently hold your hand as well, noticing the differences in how that feels.

(Exercise continues next page)

- **Noticing any emotions or thoughts:** As you observe your hand, you are invited to notice any emotions or thoughts that arise. Perhaps a memory is triggered by a scar or a piece of jewelry. Simply acknowledge these thoughts and emotions without bias or judgment, and then gently return your attention to the sensations in your hand.

- **Connecting to daily life:** Consider including a moment or two of "hand sensation awareness" in your daily activities—holding a warm cup of coffee, turning a doorknob, typing on a keyboard. Notice the sensations in your hands during these activities.

- **Gently concluding the practice:** When you're ready, you are invited to gently release your hand and with a mindful breath or two or three, gently return your attention to your surroundings.

Modifications for Limited Mobility:

Comfort and ease are key. If raising or moving your hand is difficult, you can rest it comfortably on a surface, such as your lap or a table. You can still bring your awareness to the sensations present, even without movement. If touching your hand with your other hand is challenging, you can simply focus on the sensations within the hand itself or the sensations of where your hand is in contact with its support surface. If focusing on the sensations is difficult, you could choose to focus on a different body sensation such as the feeling of your feet on the ground or the feeling of your breath moving in and out of your body.

Gently Expanding the Practice:

If you're so inclined, there are a couple of ways to gently expand this practice. The first is to simply repeat the exploration with the other hand, noticing any differences in sensations or experiences between your two hands. The second approach is to extend the duration of the practice, spending more time exploring each part of the hand. You might also try bringing mindful awareness to your hands throughout the day, noticing the sensations as you engage in various activities. No matter which approach you choose, the important point is to go at your own pace. Once again, more explorations are not "better"—it's far more valuable to be fully present with a single hand than to rush through multiple explorations without full attention. The incremental baby steps and small "wins" are our friends!

III. Concluding Chapter 3:

The simple exercises we just outlined offer a taste of how easy and simple working with mindfulness can be. Whether it's gently directing your attention to your breath, exploring your local soundscape, or exploring body sensations, using these simple approaches is an easy way to start your mindfulness journey. Remember, to be gentle with yourself when trying these exercises... there's no right or wrong way to do them and no right or wrong way to feel. Simply allow these exercises to naturally unfold. Even a few mindful moments throughout your day can make a big and positive difference in your life.

IV. Next, Chapter 4:

Now that you've considered and hopefully tried one or more of these foundational mindful moments, you're ready to expand your explorations with slightly longer techniques (but nothing too demanding). In Chapter 4, I will gently build upon the simple mindful moment exercises we just presented, and offer a few new techniques and tips to help you engage mindfulness in the ways that suit your needs and fit you best.

Chapter 4

"Be curious, not judgemental."

Walt Whitman

"The important thing is not to stop questioning.
Curiosity has its own reason for existing."

Albert Einstein

"We shall not cease from exploration,
and the end of all our exploring
will be to arrive where we started
and know the place for the first time."

T.S. Eliot

CHAPTER LEVEL TABLE OF CONTENTS

Chapter 4: Gently Leaning into Mindfulness

Chapter 4

Gently Leaning into Mindfulness

OK, now we get to build on those simple mindfulness moments we explored in the last chapter. Let's dive a little deeper in this chapter where we invite you to add to the foundation you've built and explore a few more ways to bring a gentle focus, calm, and intention into your everyday life.

I. A Quick Review & Gathering Momentum

In the last chapter, we dipped our toes into the world of mindful moments, exploring some simple ways to bring present moment awareness into everyday activities. We played with focusing on a single breath, a single object, a single taste, a single sound, and even one hand—discovering how even a simple intention and a few moments of focused attention can give rise to a sense of greater physical, mental, and emotional clarity and ease, and allow the richness of our ordinary world to shine through. Next, let's move foreward with a set of slightly longer and broader exercises.

(Exercises start next page)

II. Four More Easy Mindful Exercises

Don't worry, just relax and enjoy: Personally, I think the following four "simple" exercises are not only enjoyable, but super easy too! We invite you to drop any anxiety you have about them and just give it a go...

Exercise One: Just Ten Breaths

Our breath is an amazing constant companion—always with us, yet so often overlooked and taken for granted without a thought or care. This simple exercise invites you to reconnect with your breath, turning your attention inward to fully experience both its natural rhythm and the sensations it creates in your body. It's a wonderful way to anchor yourself in the present moment, cultivate a sense of calm and stillness, savor a peaceful moment, or even give yourself a little "reset" if you're feeling a bit off-center, agitated or ill-at-ease.

The Exercise: An Invitation to Explore

Getting ready: Find a comfortable position, either sitting, lying down, or standing. You can gently close your eyes if that feels comfortable, or keep them softly focused on a point in front of you.

- **Getting your focus:** Gently shift your awareness to your breath. Notice the sensation of the air flowing in and out of your body through your mouth or nostrils.

You don't need to change your breath in any way; simply observe it as it is.

• **Noticing the sensations:** Notice the gentle rise and fall of your chest or abdomen, changes in your mouth or lips, or the movement in your shoulders as you breathe.

• **Keeping your focus:** As you breathe in, you might silently say to yourself, "in." As you breathe out, you might silently say to yourself, "out." This can help to anchor your attention to the present moment. (Optional)

• **Returning to the breath:** If your mind wanders— and it likely will—gently guide your attention back to your breath. There's no need to judge yourself for getting distracted; simply acknowledge the wandering thought and gently return to your breath.

• **Ending and returning to your activities:** After your ten breaths, pause, noticing the sensations in your body once again, allowing those sensations to ease while you return your awareness to your surroundings. Slowly return to your normal activities.

You can return to this simple breath awareness exercise anytime you need a moment of calm and focus.

Modifications:

• If you find it difficult to follow the breath, try focusing on a more tangible sensation, such as the feeling of the air passing through your nostrils or across your lips or any other shift in your body as you breathe.

• If you experience any anxiety or discomfort during the exercise, shorten the duration to a few breaths. or focus on a grounding sensation, such as the feeling of your feet on the floor or the weight of body pressed into the chair.

Taking It Further:

• You might find it helpful to silently count your breaths. This can help further anchor your attention and can also be used to extend the exercise by increasing the count (e.g., to 20 breaths).

• If you prefer to practice for a longer period, you can extend the exercise to up to 5 minutes, following the same instructions (without counting).

• Setting a timer (with a gentle end-of-session chime or sound) can be helpful to keep track of the time, especially for longer sessions.

• You can engage in this simple breathing exercise anytime you want to take a time out to relax or simply savor any situation you are enjoying.

Exercise Two: Just Ten Steps

Movement is everywhere, isn't it? From the smallest movements within our bodies—the beating of our hearts, the flow of our breath—to all the ways we move through and interact with the world, it's a constant, incredibly complex dance, that for the most part, is done on autopilot. With this simple exercise, we invite you to bring your mindful attention to just one everyday movement—walking—and transform it into a rich and savored experience that enlivens both mind and body. It's a fantastic way to connect with your body, activate your senses, and even discover new dimensions of your balance and posture. Let's get started...

The Exercise: An Invitation to Explore

Choose your space: Find a safe space where you can take a few steps, either back and forth or even side-to-side, indoors or outdoors.

- **Start with standing:** Begin by standing still for a moment, noticing the sensations in your body—the feeling of your feet on the ground, the sense of solidity of your body, and any sensations, including tension or ease.

- **The first step:** When you're ready, take your first step. Notice the sensation of your foot leaving the ground, lifting, and then move forward to the ground again. Notice how your sense of balance shifts, how your body sensations change, how the sense of "standing still" is different from the sense of movement.

- **More steps:** Continue to either take one step at a time, or take one step after another. Moving slowly and deliberately, paying attention to each step.

(Exercise continues next page)

Besides noticing your shifting weight and balance, also allow the awareness of your leg movement and the sensations in your feet and ankles to arise. Notice too how other parts of your body are also moving, such as your arms, hands, head and neck.

• **Expanding your awareness:** As you walk, you might bring your awareness to other sensations, such as the air on your skin, the sounds around you, or the sights in your environment. But remember to keep your primary focus on the sensations of walking as much as you are able to.

• **Ending and returning to your activities:** After ten steps, pause, noticing the sensations in your body once again, allow those sensations to ease and return to your still standing awareness. Then with a few calm mindful breaths, gently allow your awareness to return to your surroundings, and then return to your normal activities.

Engage this simple exercise anytime you need some calm or simply want to enjoy the richness of your movement.

Modifications:

• If you have difficulty walking, you can adapt this exercise to other forms of movement, such as gentle swaying or rocking.

• You can also apply this approach to bicycling, an assistive scooter that uses your legs to propel it or other free-wheeling mobility device.

- If you use an assistive walking device, or even wheelchair, this exercise can be adapted easily to whatever means of movement you use, including when a caregiver is assisting you.

- If you find it difficult to focus on the sensations of walking, try focusing on a specific aspect, such as the feeling of your feet making contact with the ground, or just paying attention to your balance.

- If walking is difficult as a series of steps, try pausing after each step to regain your balance or gather your intention for the next step(s)

- If 10 steps are too many, you can start with 1 or two, and then progress as you are able to do so.

Taking It Further:

- You can extend this exercise by walking for a longer distance or time, maintaining your mindful awareness.

- Try varying your pace—walking slower or faster—and noticing how this changes the sensations in your body.

- You can also practice mindful walking in different environments, such as on a sidewalk, on a patch of grass, on a dirt path, or even in your own home. Any place you walk it a good place to try "just 10 steps."

Exercise Three: Mindful Morning Beverage

There's something special about that first cup of coffee or tea. This exercise invites you to transform this cherished ritual into a mindful experience. Think about it: For many of us, that first cup of coffee or tea is a cherished part of our day. But how often do we truly savor it—the aroma, the warmth, the taste, the entire experience? This exercise invites you to bring mindful awareness to the entire experience—from the aroma of the brewing beverage to the warmth of the cup in your hands and the taste of that first sip. By slowing down and engaging all your senses, you can transform this familiar activity into a time of deep enjoyment, connection with your senses, and even lend a touch of magic to this enjoyable part of your day. So, let's get started...

The Exercise: An Invitation to Explore

Creating a mindful environment: Before you begin, you might create a quiet and peaceful environment, free from distractions as much as is reasonably possible. Consider putting away your phone, turning off the television or radio, and adjusting the lighting to something comfortable.

• **Mindful preparation:** If you're preparing your beverage yourself, you might bring mindful awareness to each step of the process. For instance, if making coffee, you might notice the sound and smell of the beans as you grind them, the heft of the tea pot as you pur the water over the ground coffee, or the rising steam and rich aroma as the coffee brews. If making tea, you might notice the feeling of the tea leaves or bag in your hand, the sound of the water as it boils, and the changes in the water as the tea steeps and brews.

• **Choosing your cup:** You are invited to choose a cup or mug that you enjoy holding. Notice its weight, texture, and its coolness in your hands before you pour your hot beverage.

• **Holding the cup with your morning beverage:** As you hold the cup, notice its warmth, and its heft. Notice how it feels in your hands and how your hands hold the cup or mug and how they must work to keep it level and move it to your your lips.

• **Observing the beverage:** Before taking your first sip, take a moment to observe the beverage. Notice the richness of its color, the steam rising from the surface, the subtle movement of the beverage in the cup or mug, the surface of the beverage, and the warm, moist aromas that arise.

• **Taking the first sip:** Bring the cup to your lips and take a small, mindful slow sip. Notice the initial temperature of the beverage as it touches your lips and tongue. Notice the taste and texture of the first sip. Notice if any bodily sensations that arise during that first sip.

(Exercise continues next page)

• **Savoring the taste:** Allow the beverage to rest on your tongue for a moment, savoring the flavors. Notice how the taste changes as it spreads through your mouth and and it then swallow. Notice how the aromas and the tastes linger and change with time.

• **Mindful pause/breath (optional):** You might take a mindful pause here, either continuing to hold the cup or mug, setting it down for a moment and then taking one slow, conscious breath. Notice how you feel, any state of calm, joy or anticipation of the next sip. Notice the sensations of the breath entering and leaving your body.

• **Continuing to sip and savor:** You are invited to continue enjoying your beverage slowly and mindfully, noticing the changing temperature and flavors with each sip. Notice the warmth spreading through your body, the sensations of ease and enjoyment, and any feelings of relaxed contentment or joy.

• **Noticing thoughts and emotions:** As you enjoy your beverage, you are invited to notice any thoughts or emotions that arise. Simply observe them with a relaxed awareness, simply noticing them without bias or agenda, gently returning your attention to the sensations of drinking.

• **Another Mindful pause/breath (optional):** You might choose to take another mindful pause or breath at any point during the exercise, especially if you notice your mind wandering or if you simply want to deepen your connection with the present moment.

• **Finishing your beverage:** As you finish your beverage, you are invited to notice the lingering warmth and taste. The shift in your awareness as you enjoy the last sips. Take a moment or two to calmly revel in the entirety of the experience.

• **Returning to your activities:** When you're ready, take a mindful breath or two, and then gently return your attention to your surroundings, and then with intention, shift to the awareness of your day and activities.

You can engage in this mindful exercise anytime you want to bring a fuller and richer awareness to any beverage or meal you want.

Modifications for Limited Mobility:

Comfort and ease are key to this mindful experience.

• If sitting in a standard chair is uncomfortable, you can practice this exercise while sitting in a recliner with the back upright, or in a chair with good armrests and back support. You could also use pillows or cushions to support your back and arms.

• If holding a cup is difficult or if movement is limited, you can use a travel mug with a secure lid.

• If are unable to manage a hot or warm morning beverage, you can use any morning beverage either cold or room temperature, either drinking as you normally would or use a straw.

Simply follow the instructions in a way that is relevant to the beverage and way you need or want to enjoy it.

Taking It Further:

• Once you're comfortable with this mindful beverage experience, you might expand it to include a similar approach to your snacks or even full meals with focusing on the textures and aromas of your food, the sounds of chewing, or the sensations in your body as you eat.

• You might also experiment with different beverages, paying attention to the unique sensory qualities of each. For example, you could explore the subtle flavors of herbal tea, the refreshing coolness of iced water, the bubbly sensation of soda, or the rich texture of a milkshake. The possibilities are endless.

The key is to approach each experience with wide open senses, a relaxed mind, a gentle curiosity, allowing yourself to fully savor the experience.

Exercise Four: Just Relax—Head & Face

Ah, the world of tension... it seems to show up everywhere in our lives, right? We can sense it in our thoughts, feel it in our emotions, and, of course, experience in our bodies, so often carrying our tension without even realizing it. You may be surprised to learn that one of the places we frequently hold this tension is in our face and head. Think about it... it's pretty common to see a furrowed brow, a clenched jaw, pursed lips, and more—and perhaps even worn them ourselves. This simple exercise invites you to bring mindful awareness and gentle touch to the areas of your face and head, exploring tension and hopefully releasing it, and then enjoying a renewed sense of ease and calm.

First, we invite you to rest in a comfortable position. For this exercise, we recommend a seated or laying position with your head resting comfortably. **You might choose to gently close your eyes.** (Closing your eyes is optional, but closing your eyes can help you focus inward, but it's perfectly fine to keep them open if you prefer.)

• **Relax and Get Comfortable:** In a comfortable position, with your head resting against a pillow or headrest, take a slow, mindful breath or two and gently bring your awareness to your face and head. Notice any sensations of tightness or tension in your jaw, forehead, brow, eyes, or scalp.

(Exercise continues next page)

Notice the sensations of pressure and weight where your head rests against any supporting surface.

• **Begin to explore:** With either one or two hands, slowly and gently begin to explore each area of your face and head, noticning the contours and textures, any sense of heat or coolness, tension or ease.

• **Massage the tension you find:** Once you've found an area of tension, first bring your awareness to that area. Do you only notice the tension when you touch it, or is there a feeling of tension that is there even when you are not touching it?

• **Use fingers or hands:** We invite you to place either one or both hands or one or two fingers to the area and gently apply light pressures without movement.

• **Gentle touch:** Notice if the tension releases and increases as you apply your gentle touch. If it feels as though you would enjoy it, we invite you to slowly begin to massage the area with your fingertips, using comfortable slow and small circular motions.

• **Breathe:** As you massage your area of tension, take several mindful, easy deep breaths to encourage any tension release. Continue to massage this area until you feel the need to stop.

• **Massaging other areas:** If you are so inclined, move from one area of tension to another—your temples, jaw, brown, eyes, scalp, or ears—continuing the gentle slow circular massage and mindful breathing, noticing any tension release or other sensations that arise.

• **Completing your face and head explorations and massage:** Once you feel you have finished your explorations and massage, bring your awareness back to your face and head, noticing any changes. Do you sense any greater ease or comfort? Any sense or surprise about the tension? Was there any awareness of a way tension affects how your facial structure or expression?.

• **Returning to your activities:** Take a few slow, mindful deep breaths, noticing the shift in your awareness as you return to the awareness of your surroundings and begin to shift your intention to returning to any activities you want or need to engage.

You can return to this simple exercise anytime you feel tension building in your head and face or simply want to cultivate a moment of relaxation.

Modifications:

• If you experience any pain or discomfort during the massage, stop immediately and simply focus on the sensations without touch.

• If you have any skin conditions or sensitivities, adjust the massage to be very gentle or omit the massage altogether, focusing solely on awareness either with or without gentle touch.

(Modifications continue next page)

• If you are unable to reach your own face, a caregiver can perform the gentle touch and massage, respecting your comfort level.

Taking It Further:

• If you only focused on your face, you can extend this exercise by including other areas of the head and neck, such as the scalp, ears, or neck muscles, or other areas you haven't yet explored.

• You can also incorporate facial massage tools or heat/cold packs as part of your head and face relaxation routine or use facial massage tools you find comforting.

• Try combining this exercise along with the 10-Breath Awareness exercise to deepen the relaxation experience.

III. Concluding Chapter 4:

These slightly longer mindfulness explorations offer additional ways for you to connect with your breath, movement, senses, and body. By exploring and engaging with these techniques at whatever pace and level you are comfortable with, you're not only cultivating your ability to rest in present moment awareness, but also developing some valuable skills for self-care, stress reduction, and enhanced life contentment. Remember, the journey of mindfulness is a gentle process, so be patient with yourself, embrace the moment, allow any negative self talk or doubt to simply melt away, and celebrate your small wins on your journey of mindfulness.

IV. Getting Ready for Chapter 5:

In Chapter 5, I will be going into greater detail about mindfulness in general, including the 3 Pillars of Mindfulness, and highlighting how mindfulness is a flexible and powerful personal tool and some specific ways you can effectively incorporate it into your life. I will also be presenting 4 new exercises, each with two purposes and approaches... one purpose will be with focus on small discomforts or challenges, and the approach will foster an appreciation of your current activity or locations, with an emphasis on savoring and enjoying the your situation.Finally, I will introduce and do a deep dive into visualization, covering the what and why, as well as the benefits, and, of course, presenting several visualization exercises for you to try.

Chapter 5

"The little things? The little moments?
They aren't little."

Jon Kabat-Zinn

"Mindfulness isn't difficult,
we just need to remember to do it."

Sharon Salzberg

"The present moment is filled
with joy and happiness.
If you are attentive, you will see it."

Thich Nhat Hanh

CHAPTER LEVEL TABLE OF CONTENTS

Chapter 5: Expanding Your Mindfulness Toolkit

Chapter 5

Expanding Your Mindfulness Toolkit

Relax and get ready:

This chapter is long and a bit of a circuitous weave. As it meanders, it ties what has been previously presented to some new ideas and several expanded exercises, preparing us for the final chapters ahead. I recommend taking it slow; there's a lot to consider and absorb... but don't worry, I have your back and have done what I can to make the information useful and easy to understand..

I. Introduction: From Mindful Moments to Life's Ups and Downs

Think back to those quiet moments of mindful breathing, the gentle awareness of a single taste, or the simple act of noticing the world around you. In those brief experiences, you've begun to cultivate a powerful skill: present-moment awareness. As discussed earlier, mindfulness encompasses more than just individual moments. It's about uncovering a refreshed perspective, experiencing a gentler way of relating to ourselves and our experiences, increasingly free from the pressures of a critical mind, openly aware, and responding to perceptions in a way that allows us the freedom to choose responses that align with our self-envisioning. It's about recognizing and familiarizing ourselves that the present moment is the only moment we truly have access to... the only time available to us—allowing us to experience and savor life in all its complexity and richness, unfolding right here and now. Mindfulness is a tool that can help us gently step outside of our habitual mental patterns and emotional loops to meet, embrace, navigate, and even savor what unfolds before us.

Mindfulness is, as I've mentioned, very much like a toolkit—but like any toolkit, it's only useful if we actually use what's inside. And it's through using that toolkit that we are able to more easily navigate life's inevitable ups and downs without becoming derailed.

You've already been introduced to some of the essential and foundational mindfulness building blocks, or "essential tools," in that kit—present-moment awareness for our breath, sensory experiences, and body movement. You've learned how to use and directly experience these approaches as a way to anchor yourself in the here and now, to observe your thoughts and feelings without getting carried away by them, and to approach your experiences with a gentle curiosity in the spirit of self-inquiry and self-care and kindness.

Here, in this chapter, together we are building an important bridge, a bridge that connects those foundational practices and broadens the application of mindfulness to those times when life gets a little bumpy. As we move from these initial

explorations and into addressing specific situations—
ranging from everyday minor emotional ups and downs
to life's most significant challenges and transitions—you'll
see how, by using your mindfulness toolkit regularly (at
whatever level you are comfortable with), the effectiveness
and your confidence in the tools you adopt will grow and
mature.

This chapter prepares you for two things;the next chapter
on visualization (Chapter 6), as well as the three chapters
that follow (Chapters 7, 8, and 9), **where we explore in-
depth how mindfulness can support you through
some of life's most challenging situations:**

- Meeting and working with our most difficult and
upsetting emotions

- Working directly with pain and discomfort

- Navigating our experiences with grief, loss, and all the
various kinds of life transitions we encounter.

These are important and significant topics, and it's natural
to approach them with a mix of apprehension and curiosity.
But remember, you've already taken the important first
steps in learning about, experiencing, and trying several
simple yet effective mindfulness tools.

The goal is to help you refine and explore new aspects
of your mindful experience, revealing more strategies
and approaches that will prepare you for the next steps,

A deeper dive into the practical applications of mindfulness.

As you gently move into this and the following chapters, please remember that the foundational exercises are always there for you. Feel free to revisit them whenever you need a refresher, a momentary reset, or simply want to dive a little deeper into some of the mindful techniques presented. These foundational approaches are the bedrock of your mindfulness toolkit, which can be especially helpful when navigating the challenging emotions and situations we all face from time to time.

II. The Foundation of Your Mindfulness Toolkit for Life's Challenges

Now, let's put things into a broader context. The mindfulness approaches you've explored... While they work well as standalone techniques, understand that, when seen and approached as an integrated and synergistic whole, they can be a profound tool for personal transformation, both in how we experience our lives and how we interact and respond to the world. Each pillar is part of a unified whole, informing and feeding the others, both individually and collectively, to create a stable foundation for navigating our life's ups, downs, twists, and turns. Let's now turn our attention to examining how these core principles function as our mindfulness foundation—what we refer to as:

The 3 Pillars of Your Mindfulness Toolkit.

The first pillar is the heart of mindfulness: Simple awareness—a clear sense of what's happening in the present moment. This present-moment awareness is cultivated through choosing to focus or gently nudge our attention to our direct present moment experience, whether that's the breath, our body's sensations, our movements, our senses taking in the world, as well as our thoughts and emotions.

But let's be clear... mindfulness is not about emptying the mind or stopping our thoughts. Rather, it's about observing the totality of our perceived experience a with a degree of calmness and a relaxed curiosity, much like resting and watching clouds floating by, without getting caught up in the stories, thoughts, or emotions that arise. This present-moment awareness is our first step toward a calmer response and tempering our emotional flare-ups.

When we are able to maintain some present-moment awareness as strong emotions arise, we are better equipped to meet them and, in time, ride their undulations without being derailed or swept out to sea.

Next, let's look at the second pillar: Kindness and acceptance. These two sides of the same coin—a linked kindness-acceptance coin, if you will—make an important contribution to our mindfulness practice, helping us stabilize our present-moment awareness.

Kindness, both to ourselves and others, allows us to approach experiences with tenderness and caring, recognizing that we all struggle in one way or another. Suffering, in large and small ways, is a universal part of our shared human experience.

Acceptance allows us to simply acknowledge "what is," or what is being currently experienced, without resistance or judgment (even if that resistance or judgment is what is arising!). It's a calm abiding, an interim non-agenda openness to what is unfolding in our experience. We are simply witnessing what has arisen (this is not to be interpreted as a continual or extended state of "no action" when action is needed).

By understanding how the kindness/acceptance tool functions—rather than simply paying lip service to these terms—we can begin to sense their potential to unlock our calm and release our agitated states. Seeing the kindness/acceptance duo as a single multi-functional tool is key.

Acceptance softens the sharp edges of difficult emotions, while kindness creates a safe space to be with, and even explore, those emotions. Together, these complementary qualities allow us to experience and express a natural compassion, both for ourselves and others. By gently allowing kindness and acceptance to arise, we build a functional resilience with the capacity to embrace, grow, and learn from each challenge.

The final pillar is curiosity: While curiosity is often understood as a trait related to our approach and investigation of the world, in our mindfulness journey, **curiosity is seen as a tool of gentle self-inquiry** *(and definitely not a critical or judgmental self-inquiry).*

Curiosity fuels our present-moment awareness explorations. It allows us to approach each moment with wonder—like a scientist making discoveries—gaining new insights about ourselves, the world, and our relationship to everything we experience. Curiosity helps us stay engaged with the present, even when it's challenging and uncomfortable! It is also an important ingredient for building mental and emotional resilience. When we approach challenges with calm curiosity, we are more likely to perceive and experience them directly. We see them not as threats or personal attacks, but as opportunities for growth, learning, and even enjoyment.

These core three pillars—awareness, kindness/acceptance, and curiosity—are the fundamental ingredients of our mindfulness toolkit. Let's explore how they work together to create a flexible, easy-to-use, and adaptable resource.

Mindfulness as a Toolkit for Life

Our mindfulness toolkit is a functional and robust personal raft for life's whitewater rapids. It keeps us out of harm's way, afloat when things get rough, and cushions the blows when we encounter submerged rocks.

And just as a hammer is designed for specific tasks, each mindfulness technique serves a purpose within this functional toolkit.

For example, breath awareness can anchor us when we feel overwhelmed. Mindful body movement can lower the heat of emotions when we are upset and help release agitation. Sensory exploration can reconnect us to the present and help release tension, returning us to a calmer state. Another example, if we're anxious before a presentation, a few mindful breaths can help regulate emotions and approach the situation with greater calm, clarity, and focus.

Mindfulness is also a reliable toolkit. The mindfulness approaches are grounded in time-honored traditions and cultures. Even today, these techniques are known to be effective in reducing stress, managing emotions, and cultivating well-being. Like any well-crafted tool, they are designed to work consistently and reliably when used with intention and some basic knowledge. Whether it's breathing, movement, or body sensations, they are a reliable way to release mental knots, emotional flare-ups, and physical tensions.

The mindfulness toolkit is readily available. Whether it's our breath, our senses, or our ability to move, we can bring awareness to any activity or situation. These portable, accessible tools are ready to be used whenever and wherever we need them. Whether it's a few mindful moments or a longer engagement with a taste, a sound, or a sensation, we can experience a calming shift in our approach and perceptions even during a difficult task, an upsetting day, or a challenging life event.

While simple, this mindfulness toolkit empowers us to meet and embrace the challenges that life places in our path. As we become more familiar with these tools and techniques, we reinforce our mental calm and emotional resilience.

Engaging the three pillars—awareness, kindness/ acceptance, and curiosity—develops our capacity to respond to difficult emotions and situations with greater wisdom, ease, clarity, calm, and compassion. We move beyond reacting with unchecked thought habits, emotional patterns, and repeated "personal story" loops.

This flexible framework is resilient to life's storms, allowing us to learn from our missteps, adapt to change, and maintain equilibrium, whether facing adversity or savoring life's joys.

III. Chapter 5 Exercises

Expanding Your Toolkit With Several New Exercises: Preparing for the Journey Ahead

For this first exercise "Just Breathe", it's important to first reconnect with the foundational techniques of breath awareness presented in Chapters 3 and 4, exploring how even a single mindful breath can bring calm and focus.

Now, we'll delve deeper into this effective and powerful tool, exploring how extended periods of breath awareness can cultivate a profound connection to your inner world, enhance your capacity for emotional regulation, and even add a new found depth to your appreciation of life.

This next extended breath awareness exploration has two options: one is to use your breath to navigate challenging moments, and the second is to use your breath to enjoy and savor the situation you are in.

While the initial foundational breath exercises offered a taste of mindfulness, these expanded explorations provide opportunities to develop your concentration, deepen your understanding of the mind-body connection, and build greater resilience to the winds of change and emotional upset.

Now, let's get started with our Chapter 5 exercises. *(For those interested in more structured breath-focused meditations or exercises, there are many excellent resources available by other authors.):*

Exercise 1: Just Breathe—A Deeper Dive into Breath Awareness

This exploration invites you to connect with your breath in a way that best serves your needs or inclinations in the moment. Whether you need to engage these approaches for a moment or two, or an extended time, there is no "time constraint" that you need to adhere to. By simply "breathing" with mindful awareness you can use this approach to either reset an emotional upset you are experiencing or simply to savor and enjoy the place or situation that you find in.

Exercise 1 - Option 1:
Breath as a Tool for Calming Upset

When you find yourself feeling stressed, anxious, or emotionally overwhelmed, your breath can be a powerful anchor.

- **Find a comfortable or balanced position** (sitting, standing, or even walking slowly, and potentially someplace away from the source of the upset).

- **Bring your awareness to your breath.** Notice the sensation of the air flowing in and out of your body, whether it is the rise and fall of the abdomen or chest, the air passing through your nostrils, or over your lips.

(Exercise continues next page)

Change your breath in any way that helps you regain your calm. (Slow full deep breaths with a slight force behind the exhale with lightly pursed lips is one technique. Simple gentle breathing is another)

• **Just watch and observe your breath.** If the upset is large, once you have calmed a bit, just begin to observe your breath as it is, without trying to change or alter it in any way. It's okay if it's fast or shallow; rapid or slow, simply notice it as it is, and to the degree you are able, pay very close attention to every aspect of the breath that you can follow and observe.

• **As you breathe,** if you are so inclined, you gently remind yourself that you are safe (assuming that you are in a safe location) and that this feeling and upset will soon pass. You can repeat this reminder silently to yourself with each breath if you find it helpful.

• **Continue focusing on your breath** until you feel a shift in your emotional state and you feel a return of your emotional well-being and re-balancing.

• **Gently return your awareness to your surroundings.**

Exercise 1 - Option 2:
Breath for Savoring the Moment

Your breath can also be a wonderful way to fully connect with and appreciate your surroundings or activities in the present moment.

- **Moving or at rest, pause in mindful awareness** settling into a state of comfort and ease.

- **Slowly take in a series of gentle breaths**, keeping a soft focus on your breath while gently noticing your surroundings with eyes open with a soft focus, or closed as you see fit.

- **Notice the subtle sensations of relaxation and enjoyment** that rise and fall with each breath you take.

- **Allow yourself to relax** and be fully present with your surroundings and the rhythm of your breath, savoring the situation and location and the breath.

- **Continue this exploration** for as long as you feel comfortable doing so.

- **Gently return your awareness to the activities you were engaged in.**

Remember, there's no right or wrong way to engage with your breath. The key is to approach it with a gentle acceptance, kindness, and curiosity, allowing it to carry you into a sense of great ease, calm, and connection.

Exercise 2: Just Move—Mindful Motion

Just as your breath can be a powerful anchor, mindful movement offers another way to connect with your body, thoughts, and emotions, as well as the present moment.

This set of exercises invites you to bring awareness to your movements, whether it's a gentle stretch, a mindful walk, or simply noticing the sensations as you go about your day.

Mindful activity can be a valuable tool for releasing tension, reducing stress, and easing anxiety, as well as calming emotional upheavals. Movement helps us cultivate a deeper understanding of our body's signals, alerting us to mental and emotional imbalances.

But movement doesn't have to be limited to a formal activity such as yoga, tai chi, or "mindful walking"; it can include any activity you enjoy, such as golfing, swimming, riding a bike, or even having a picnic.

Movement is a wonderful way to integrate mindfulness into every activity, transforming our ordinary daily movements into opportunities for connection, self-discovery, and even gratitude and joy.

Exercise 2 - Option 1:
Mindful Movement for Releasing Tension

When you're feeling stressed, tight, anxious, or emotionally overwhelmed, mindful movement can help you release physical tension and upsets and also allow for new perspectives and insights to emerge while also resetting and restoring your mental and emotional equilibrium.

- **First, find a comfortable space** where you can move freely and safely. (Be sure to accommodate any body limitations you may have.)

- **Begin with some very gentle movements** or easy stretches. Start to explore the range of your motions. Notice the different sensations in your body as you slowly move and shift. There is no need to rush, push, or strain; simply notice how your body feels, the range of your limbs, the smoothness of your movement, the comfort or discomfort that arises, or any other sensation that you become aware of.

- **As you mindfully explore your body's movements,** allow your awareness to flow into the parts of your body that feel tense, tight, or sore. Breathe gently as you move those areas, noticing any changes in those sensations. (You can also try "breathing into your tension" and then with each out-breath "releasing the tension.")

- **Explore different types of movement,** such as swaying, rotating, shifting your balance from foot to foot, stretching, or even moving from sitting to standing. The key is to move with an easy and gentle awareness, always

(Exercise continues next page)

listening to your body and respecting its limits, paying attention to both the subtle and not-so-subtle sensations in your body. Pay attention to your body's structures, such as muscles and joints, as well as your balance and your mental state.

• **Continue your mindful movement exploration** for as long as it feels helpful, comfortable, and easy, noticing how your body sensations change as you move and the tension begins to release.

• **Gently return your awareness to the activities you were engaged in.**

Exercise 2 - Option 2:
Mindful Movement in Everyday Life

It's important to understand that mindful movement isn't just about formal relaxation exercises or specific outlined regimens. You can bring present-moment awareness to any movement and any activity, large or small, easy or hard, familiar or new.

• **As you go about your day, choose an activity to focus on,** such as walking, washing dishes, writing in a journal, or even typing on your computer.

• **Bring your attention to the sensations in your body as you perform this activity.** Notice the movement of your muscles, the feeling of your feet on the ground, the subtle shifts in your posture, and the way your body's balance comes into play.

• **Allow yourself to be fully present with the experience of both the large and small movements,** noticing any connections you sense between your thoughts, feelings, and physical sensations.

• **Continue your mindful movement explorations throughout your day**, either for a set time, number of steps or breaths, or as you feel inclined. Notice how bringing your awareness of the present moment enhances and deepens your appreciation of your experiences, even for the most mundane and ordinary tasks.

Exercise 2 - Option 3: Mindful Movement for Joy and Gratitude

As many of us know, movement can be a source of great joy and contentment and often lead to feelings of both physical and mental relaxation. Movement can also give rise to feelings of joy, deep appreciation, and even awe. This movement exploration invites you to engage in any activity that you like to do, as a way to connect you to the positive and joy-filled side of your mindfulness adventures.

• **Choose a movement or activity that you enjoy,** whether it's dancing, hiking, swimming, playing tennis, or any other form of movement that brings a smile to your heart.

(Exercise continues next page)

• **As you start or continue your activity,** bring your attention to the sensations in your body, and notice the feelings of freedom, energy, or lightness as they become apparent.

• **Allow yourself to fully experience the wonders,** pleasures, and sense of joy that arise from fully experiencing your body's movements. Revel in the synergy and amazing ways you are able to interact with and move through the world.

• **If you feel so inclined,** add gratitude to the activity. Relish in the richness of moving. Smile and rejoice in the act of movement. Savor this awareness and connection with your body. Be kind to yourself as you move, recognizing and appreciating all that your body can do.

• **Continue this exploration for as long as it feels comfortable and joy-filled,** allowing yourself to fully experience and even express in words or movement all your feelings. Be filled with awe and wonder as you interact with your surroundings.

Remember, there's no right or wrong way to engage with mindful movement. Simply be authentic with your movements, no matter how modest or grand. The key is to approach it with as much present-moment awareness as you can, a sense of joy and gratitude, remembering to be kind and curiously inquisitive, resting in a state of greater ease, sense of connection, self-understanding, and deep appreciation for the joy and miracle of movement.

Exercise 3: Just Be—Everyday Mindfulness

Remember, mindfulness isn't just about formal practices (though you can certainly engage a more formal approach if you want to). Our approach is softer. We simply want to encourage you to use mindfulness as a tool as YOU see fit and feels right for your circumstances and personal preferences. In other words, feel free to use these exercises in any part of your life that you choose, even the most ordinary moments that seem to mostly run on autopilot.

In the following two exercises, you are invited to explore two different approaches:

• The first is about bringing your mindful attention to an ordinary task in your life, paying attention to your thoughts, emotions, and bodily sensations as you engage that task.

• The second is a "non-doing" approach, where you are simply relaxed in a state of awareness without "doing" anything in particular other than noticing anything and everything that arises in any of your sense fields, including any thoughts and emotions that arise.

These two exercise options that follow are about discovering and fully experiencing the richness and depth that is present in every facet of our lives.

Exercise 3 - Option 1:
Mindful Moments in Daily Life

If you have managed to read this far in the book, you are likely aware of how much of our waking hours are performed on autopilot. Of course, this is the "efficient" way to get things done, but it is also missing the rich experiences that can be revealed in each and every moment.

This first exercise option invites you to intentionally bring your present-moment awareness to an everyday activity, slowing down, and really paying close attention to each aspect of the task you are engaged with. There is no goal, per se, other than to just "pay attention" and allow yourself to experience your world in a new way.

- **Choose an activity to focus on.** It could be anything from brushing your teeth to washing dishes, eating a meal, waiting in line, chewing gum, or even tying your shoe. Any activity you choose is OK.

- **Endeavor to "open your senses"** to all sensations, thoughts, and emotions as you perform your activity. Notice the feeling of the toothbrush in your hand and the flavor of the toothpaste, the warmth of the water on your skin and any thoughts of "too hot" or "too cold," explore the taste and texture of your food and any thoughts or emotions that arise, or simply observe your breath as you vacuum, take out the trash or recycling, or even wait in line. Simply notice these inner experiences without trying to change them, label them, or resist them.

• **Expand your awareness** to include all your senses if you can. Notice the sights, lights, and colors. Hear all the sounds that come in and out of your hearing range. Focus on the smells, tastes, and tactile sensations that accompany the activity. What colors do you see? What sounds do you hear? What aromas do you notice?

• **Connect with your inner experience.** As you engage your senses, pay attention to the thoughts and emotions that arise. Are you feeling rushed or relaxed? Are you thinking about the past or the future? Do you experience your activity as joyful or distasteful?

• **Continue this type of mindful exploration** throughout your day as you feel so inclined. Notice how it changes your sense of the world and how even the most mundane tasks and activities can take on a new depth of experience.

Exercise 3 - Option 2:
Moments of Stillness

The title for this exercise section is "Just Being," but I like to think that our experience of "being" exists within a large spectrum of variations. While most mindful techniques involve a subtle form of "doing," combined with a "being" component (ie; "I am going to do a mindfulness exercise now"), there is also an approach where we can simply be— present with ourselves and the world around us without any agenda and without any active "doing." These "moments of stillness" can be another powerful opportunity to connect and gain familiarity with our inner and outer worlds, often glossed over when we are in our "getting stuff done" mode.

- **First, find a place** (inside or outside, busy or quiet, hectic or calm, and always safe) where you can comfortably "be" for a few minutes. Your position doesn't matter; standing, sitting, or laying down are all fine, as long as you can remain still for a period of time (the amount of time is up to you and your comfort level).

- **As you enter and embody your stillness**, allow all of your senses to come alive. Let the cascade of sights, sounds, smells, and tactile sensations flood into your awareness while you remain in an easy and relaxed "still" position. Let the world carry you along on the waves of whatever is in your sphere of observation.

- **Allow yourself to simply be present** with anything that comes to you without changing a thing. Just "be" with whatever shows up.

- **Without any active "forced observing,"** continue to just allow the sensations to wash over you and then recede without any attempt to alter anything.

- **In your stillness,** thoughts and feelings may arise as well. Let them be a part of the symphony of what you are aware of. Let them be as fleeting as a bird's path across the sky. Simply observe and let the outer and inner world mingle without effort.

- **Continue this relaxed state** of "simply being gentle awareness" for as long as you are comfortable doing so.

- **Gently return to your surroundings.** When you are ready, take a mindful breath or two or three and gently return to whatever activity or task you choose.

These "being" interludes can be a wonderful way to relax and also connect with your surroundings, friends, family, as well as your inner world. This "simply being" approach will be further developed in the following "Just Relax" and "Just Enjoy" exercise sections, where we'll delve deeper into states of deep relaxation as well as exploring a world of wonderment, richness and awe.

And remember, there's absolutely no way you can do these exercises "wrong." Just engaging the exercises in whatever way or whatever level is "your way" is the perfect way for you.

There is nothing to "get right." The only thing you are doing is just resting, revealing your innate natural awareness to shine in the kaleidoscopic display of our everyday world.

And as always, approach these exercises with gentleness, an open heart, kindness, and a spirit of curiosity and inquiry, allowing whatever arises to appear and then fade into the next perception.

Exercise 4 Just Relax & Enjoy: Settling into the Present Moment

As we continue our journey along the gentle meandering path of mindfulness, it is here, dear reader, where we intentionally shift our approach with the two following exercises, and invite you to walk with us, as we take a gentle step from the shores of "a self doing stuff" into the relaxing warm pool of vast, spacious open awareness.

In these next two explorations, I will be lightly touching on the heart of "being," and glimpsing the facet of mindfulness that is more expansive, exploring two distinct yet interconnected pathways revealing a richness of our present-moment experiences.

The first approach, "Swept Away With Awe," is an invitation to savor the richness of the totality of experience, allowing ourselves to be filled with a deep appreciation, joy, and wonderment of the world just as it is, and gently resting into the amazing complexity and interconnectedness of what we perceive but cannot fully grasp.

The second approach, "Letting Go—Just Be," is an invitation to release our ideas, our solid sense of self, our fears, anxieties, tension, our clinging to notions of this and that, and our need to "do something," and "be something," allowing ourselves to effortlessly rest in the boundless spaciousness of spontaneously arising awareness. These two approaches are different faces of the same faceted jewel, allowing for an expansive sense that softens our normal points of reference, and resets our experience of "self," and the world that we experience, revealing the natural perfection of our being infused with abiding ease, joy, and calm.

Exercise 4 - Option 1:
Just Enjoy—Swept Away With Awe

In this first exploration, I invite you to savor the richness of the present moment, allowing yourself to be carried away with wonder and awe as you fully allow every sensory or mental perception you experience, whether it is the sense of an "internal" landscape filled with thoughts or emotions, or the external landscape filled with things and movement. Relaxing into the totality of perceptions, allowing joy and appreciation to arise as the grasp of identity and "this and that" is gently set aside, during your chosen place to engage our "Swept Away With Awe" exercise. I are simply encouraging you to gently release all bias, preference, or agenda and allow your inherent "wow" and "awe" to shine forth... appreciating, savoring with delighting in the ever-changing kaleidoscopic display of life, beautiful and awesome in its vastness and complexity, yet as fleeting as the wind. There is nothing to strive for here, nothing to grasp. Simply relax into the unrelenting beauty and richness that is every moment.

(Exercise starts next page)

• **First, Choose a place** where you can comfortably "be" (inside or outside, busy or quiet, hectic or calm, and always safe) for a few minutes or longer. Your position doesn't matter; standing, sitting, or lying down are all fine, as long as you can remain still and at ease, totally relaxed for a period of time (the amount of time is up to you and your comfort level).

• **As you settle into this space,** gently allow all of your senses to come alive. Let the cascade of sights, sounds, smells, and tactile sensations flood into your awareness while you remain in your easy and relaxed "still" position. Let the world carry you along on the waves of whatever is in your sphere of perception. (Alternatively, you can also explore imagined landscapes or experiences from your past). No matter your location, choose one that will support and allow for your sense of wonder, awe, appreciation, and joy to naturally arise.

• **Allow yourself to simply be present** with anything that arises in your mental or sensory perceptions without any effort or striving, without changing a thing. Just relax into "being" with whatever shows up, relaxing all mental constraints and fixed points of reference. Allow a sense of all-inclusive spaciousness to naturally arise.

• **Without any "forced observing"** on your part, continue to just allow the perceptions, feelings, thoughts, and sensations to wash over you and then recede without any attempt to alter, follow, fixate on anything.

• **In your expansive sense of stillness,** simply rest in the endlessly shifting kaleidoscopic and symphonic display. Let whatever arises be as fleeting as a bird's path across the sky. Simply rest with your senses wide open allowing the outer and inner world to effortlessly mingle.

• **Continue riding and savoring** this relaxed state of "simply being with gentle awareness" for as long as you are comfortable doing so.

• **Gently return to your surroundings.** When you are ready, take a mindful breath or two or three and gently return to whatever activity or task you choose.

This is one of my favorite exercises and one I think of as a "delicious dessert" that infuses our sense of self with joy and gratitude. I believe this "moments of awe" is a wonderful way to connect with the inherent joy and beauty that surrounds us, both within and without.

Exercise 4 - Option 2:
Just Relax: Letting Go—Just Be

In this second exploration, I invite you to relax into the boundless totality of perception, resting easy, fully content, at peace, floating along on the undulating waters of the passing world, and once again, gently releasing our notions of "this and that."

(Exercise continues next page)

In a deeply relaxed, but aware state, we allow the world of perceptions to appear and pass without a trace, leaving nothing but pure perception, revealing a foundational experience of ease and complete contentment.

Again, there is nothing to strive for here, no goal to reach, nothing to obtain, no level to achieve, nothing but a relaxed open awareness. Simply at ease, we simultaneously experience and release everything as it arises into the boundless and ungraspable present moment.

> • **Choose a place** where you can comfortably "be" (inside or outside, busy or quiet, hectic or calm, and always safe) for a few minutes or longer. Your position doesn't matter; standing, sitting, or lying down are all fine, as long as you can remain still and at ease, totally relaxed for a period of time (the amount of time is up to you and your comfort level).

> • **As you settle into this space,** gently and naturally allow all of your senses to come alive. Let the cascade of sights, sounds, smells, and tactile sensations flood into your awareness while you remain in your easy and relaxed "still" position. Let the world carry you along on the waves of whatever is in your sphere of perception. No matter your location, choose one that will support and allow for you to completely relax, giving the space for whatever perceptions arise, drift along and then simply fall away. (Note: The alternative, "explore imagined landscapes or experiences from your past" approach that

was part of the previous exercise is not appropriate for this exercise).

• **Allow yourself to simply be present** with anything that arises in your mental or sensory perceptions without any effort or striving, without changing a thing. Just relax into "being" with whatever shows up, relaxing all mental constraints and fixed points of reference. Allow a sense of all-inclusive spaciousness to naturally arise.

• **Continue to relax** without any active "forced observing", allowing the perceptions, feelings, thoughts, and sensations to simply wash over you and then recede without any attempt to alter, follow, or fixate on anything.

• **Now, deeply relaxed, but fully aware,** allow the world of perceptions to be as gossamer as an apparition, as fleeting as reflections in a mirror, as enchanting as a multicolored light show, as fanciful as the shapes in passing clouds, or as ethereal as the full moon reflected in calm waters. Allow each moment to pass without a trace, leaving nothing but pure perception, effortlessly revealing a natural sense of great ease and complete contentment.

• **Continue riding the expanded awareness.** Allow the flow of this relaxed state of "simply aware" for as long as you are comfortable doing so.

• **Gently return to your surroundings.** When you are ready, take several mindful breaths and gently return to the your normal waking world. (We recommend that you continue to rest and reorient yourself after completing this exercise, before moving on with your day)

This exercise is anotherh one of my favorites, another of the "delicious dessert" mindfulness approaches, one that I feel has the capacity to infuse our mind with a stable and deeply relaxed but aware foundation that allows us to interact with and move through the world with clarity as well as mental and emotional calm.

Conclusion for Chapter 5:
You've Built Your Mindfulness Foundation!

I hope these mindfulness exercises have been helpful. Having explored foundational mindfulness tools and techniques—from breath awareness and body scans to mindful movement—you've built a powerful foundation. Remember to revisit these practices regularly so they're readily available when you need them. Remember, these exercises are yours to personalize. Adapt them to fit your specific needs and preferences. And don't forget that mindfulness can be a way to enjoy life! It's not always about "facing challenging emotions" or working with old mental habits.

Next, in Chapter 6, we'll explore another powerful tool that complements your mindfulness practice: Visualization.

Chapter 6

"The inner landscape is as important
as the outer landscape."

Anonymous

"The world of reality has its limits;
the world of imagination is boundless."

Jean-Jacques Rousseau

"The soul never thinks without a mental picture."

Aristotle

CHAPTER LEVEL TABLE OF CONTENTS

Chapter 6: Visualization: Another Layer of Mindfulness

Chapter 6

Visualization: Another Layer of Mindfulness

I. What is Visualization?

Visualization, at its core, is the process of creating mental images or representations using our abilities to imagine and/or our ability to envision a sensory experience.

It is much more than just "seeing pictures in our head"; it can involve all or some of our senses, depending on the visualization, including sights, sounds, smells, tastes, and tactile sensations, and even weave them into dynamic inner experiences.

These mental representations can have a powerful influence on our inner perceptions and experiences. While visualization is often associated with specific outcomes (like visualizing success in sports or a desired change in life, or even a deep state of relaxation), in this book, I approach visualization as a powerful tool for deepening our connection to the present moment and cultivating a landscape of inner calm and fostering a relaxed sense of ease and well-being.

Understanding Visualization in the Context of Mindfulness: Visualization, while often considered a distinct technique, has a close relationship with both mindfulness and meditation. Here are some short general definitions to help you understand the differences:

Mindfulness: The practice of cultivating present-moment awareness, a way of being fully present with whatever arises.

Meditation: A practice frequently used to support the development of mindfulness, offering techniques to train the mind.

Visualization: The process of creating mental images or sensory experiences, can be a powerful tool within a meditation practice, enhancing focus and deepening the experience.

With these definitions in mind, it's easier to see how visualization fits into the larger picture. Here are some examples:

• One way that visualization can be used is as a guided meditation, such as a Loving-Kindness meditation, where the visualizations might incorporate images of loved ones, oneself, or even all beings.

• When visualization is used as part of a mindfulness exercise, it might involve seeing the breath as colored light flowing through the body.

• Visualization can also be a standalone practice, used to achieve specific goals like relaxation or stress reduction.

In this book, we present visualization as a valuable adjunct to mindfulness, a technique that can both deepen present-moment awareness and offer unique benefits of its own.

Purpose and Benefits of Visualization: I have introduced visualization at this stage of our exploration because it naturally builds upon the foundations we've established in the previous exercises. Just as we've explored the power and soothing aspects of breath, movement, and mindful present-moment awareness, visualization offers another avenue for connecting with an inner world that has the potential to add depth and insight into our understanding of self.

Visualization can be a powerfully effective tool for enhancing creativity and problem-solving. **It can also provide an invaluable supportive framework to help us navigate some of life's most upsetting challenges**—a theme we'll explore in much greater depth in the next three chapters.

II. Types of Visualizations

Visualizations, like mindfulness and meditation, come in a variety of forms, each offering unique benefits and experiences. Understanding these different types can help you choose the visualizations that best suit your needs and preferences.

Simple Visualizations: These visualizations focus on a single element, allowing for deep concentration and relaxation. Examples include:

• **Color Visualization:** Imagine a calming color, like a deep blue or a soft green, filling your mind's eye. Focus on the hue, the saturation, and the feeling it evokes.

• **Shape Visualization:** Visualize a simple shape, like a circle, a square, or a triangle. Explore its form, its edges, and its presence in your mind. A circle, for example, can represent wholeness or interconnectedness.

• **Object Visualization:** Choose a simple object, like a flower, a leaf, or a candle flame. Visualize it in detail, noticing its shape, color, texture, and any other sensory details that arise.

Complex Visualizations: These visualizations involve creating a more elaborate scene or scenario, engaging multiple senses and emotions. Examples include:

• **Nature Scene:** Imagine yourself walking through a peaceful forest, hearing the rustling leaves, smelling the fresh earth, and feeling the sunlight on your skin.

• **Personal Sanctuary:** Create a visualization of a place where you feel completely safe, comfortable, and at peace. This could be a real place you've visited or an imagined sanctuary.

• **Journey Visualization:** Embark on an inner journey, exploring different landscapes, encountering symbolic figures, or overcoming challenges.

Guided Visualizations: These visualizations involve following a pre-recorded script or an instructor's guidance. They can be particularly helpful for beginners or those who find it challenging to create their own visualizations. Examples include:

• **Body Scan Meditation:** A guided visualization that involves systematically focusing attention on different parts of the body, promoting relaxation and body awareness.

• **Loving-Kindness Meditation:** A guided visualization that cultivates feelings of love and compassion for oneself and others.

• **Progressive Relaxation:** A guided visualization that involves tensing and releasing different muscle groups to promote deep relaxation.

Creative/Free Visualizations: These visualizations allow for free exploration of your imagination and inner world. They can be used to explore solutions to problems, visualize desired outcomes, or simply to enhance creativity. Examples include:

Problem-Solving Visualization: Seeing yourself successfully navigating a challenging situation and the steps you might take and the positive outcome you desire.

Goal Visualization: Visualize yourself achieving a specific goal, experiencing the feelings of accomplishment and satisfaction.

Dream Exploration: Revisit a dream in your mind, exploring its imagery, emotions, and potential meanings.

Metaphorical Visualizations: These visualizations use symbolic imagery to represent abstract concepts, emotions, or experiences. They can be a powerful way to work with inner experiences and gain deeper insights. Examples include:

• **Visualizing Emotions:** Imagine anger as a storm, sadness as a gray cloud, or joy as a radiant sun.

• **Visualizing Challenges:** Imagine a challenge as a mountain to climb, a river to cross, or a maze to navigate.

• **Visualizing Personal Growth:** Imagine yourself as a seed growing into a strong tree, a caterpillar transforming into a butterfly, or a rough stone being polished into a gem.

More About Guided Visualizations: A Helpful Alternative

Visualization, while easy for many, can be challenging for some. If you find it difficult to create mental images, be patient with yourself. Allow whatever experience you have to simply be what it is, without self-criticism. There's no right or wrong way to visualize. We encourage you to experiment with different approaches.

For those who have trouble with self-guided visualizations, or for anyone wanting a different approach, we recommend guided visualizations (sometimes referred to as guided meditations). These are a viable and effective alternative or supplement, especially for beginners. Guided visualizations are available through various sources, including in-person sessions with qualified instructors, therapists, or groups, as well as through apps, audio-books, and online recordings. Finding the approach and the visualizations that resonate with you is key.

III. The Visualization Connection to Mindfulness

Visualization and mindfulness are deeply interconnected practices that enhance and support each other. Cultivating mindfulness can significantly improve your ability to visualize, while visualization, in turn, can deepen your mindfulness practice.

Mindfulness, with its emphasis on present-moment awareness and non-judgmental observation, provides a strong foundation for effective visualization. When you approach visualization with a mindful mindset, you're better able to focus your attention on the inner imagery without getting carried away by thoughts or distractions. Mindfulness helps you observe your visualizations with relaxed curiosity and non-agenda acceptance, allowing the experience to unfold naturally without striving or forcing.

Conversely, visualization can be a powerful tool for deepening your mindfulness practice. By intentionally focusing your attention on specific images, sensations, or scenarios, you strengthen your ability to concentrate and direct your awareness. Visualization can also help you explore your inner world with greater curiosity and insight, leading to a deeper understanding of your thoughts, emotions, and experiences.

Additionally, visualization itself can be considered a form of mindfulness. When you engage in visualization, you are essentially focusing your attention on your inner world, observing the images, sensations, and emotions that arise. This process of focused attention and observation is a core element of mindfulness.

Combining mindfulness and visualization has the potential to create a synergistic effect, enhancing the benefits of both practices. By cultivating the mindfulness qualities of non-biased perception, acceptance of what is, and present-moment awareness, you can create more vivid and transformative visualizations. And by using visualization to explore your inner world, you can deepen your understanding of yourself and cultivate greater self-awareness, which is a key aspect of mindfulness.

Benefits of Visualization

Visualization offers a wide range of benefits for both physical and mental well-being, including:

- Stress Reduction

- Deep Relaxation

- Pain Management

- Improved Sleep

- Emotional Regulation

- Goal Achievement

- Working with Illness and Injury.

- Life Contentment

IV. Tips for Effective Visualization

Visualization is a skill that develops with practice. While some people naturally find it easy to create mental images, others may find it more challenging. To make the most of your visualization practice, consider the following tips:

Find a Comfortable and Quiet Space: Minimize distractions by choosing a comfortable and quiet place where you can relax undisturbed for a few minutes. Turn off your phone, close the door, and let others know you need some quiet time. Consider the temperature of the room – you may want to dress warmly or have a blanket nearby, as it's common to feel cool or even shiver during visualizations, especially longer ones.

Prepare Your Environment: You may wish to use a quiet background soundtrack of nature sounds or soothing music to enhance your experience. If so, set up your sound source before you begin. Sometimes performing visualizations outdoors in a peaceful and tranquil setting can be a wonderful alternative.

Relax Your Body: Start with a few slow, deep breaths to release tension in your body. You can also incorporate gentle stretches or progressive muscle relaxation to further enhance relaxation. A relaxed body allows the mind to settle more easily. Visualizations are usually best performed either seated or lying down (face-up). If laying down, face up, a pillow under the knees can aid in leg comfort. A small pillow under the head can also ease any discomfort when laying on the floor. Laying on a pad or blanket can also help with comfort during extended visualizations. Removing glasses and wearing loose-fitting clothing can also help us relax into the visualization process.

Start Simple: If you're new to visualization, begin with simple visualizations, such as imagining a color, a shape, or a single object. As your skills develop, you can gradually progress to more complex scenes and scenarios. Don't try to create elaborate visualizations right away; start small and build from there.

Engage Multiple Senses: The more senses you involve in your visualization, the more immersive and realistic it will feel. Try to incorporate sights, sounds, smells, tastes, and tactile sensations into your mental imagery. For example, if you're visualizing a beach, imagine the sound of the waves, the smell of the salt air, and the feel of the warm sand beneath your feet.

Be Patient: Visualization takes practice. Don't get discouraged if you find it challenging at first. Some days your visualizations may be more vivid than others. The key is to be patient with yourself and to practice regularly. Even short, consistent visualization sessions can be beneficial.

Items for Enhancing Visualization: Some people find it helpful to use items to enhance their visualizations. For example, you can hold a crystal, light a candle, use aromatherapy oils, or incorporate sounds from a small gong, bell, or Tibetan singing bowl to create a more sensory-rich environment. These items can serve as anchors for your visualizations and help you focus your attention.

Simply Allow: Allow whatever images arise in your mind to come without judgment. There's no right or wrong way to visualize. If your mind wanders, gently redirect your attention back to your visualization. The goal is not to achieve perfect mental stillness, but rather to cultivate a gentle and accepting awareness of your inner world.

Practice Can Help: Like any skill, visualization improves with regular practice. Try to incorporate visualization into your daily routine, even if it's just for a few minutes each day. You can visualize first thing in the morning, before bed, or anytime you need a moment of calm and focus.

V. Visualization Themes

The possibilities for visualization themes are as vast as your imagination. However, some common themes tend to be particularly effective for promoting relaxation, well-being, and self-discovery. Here are a few examples to get you started:

Nature Scenes: Visualizing peaceful natural environments, such as mountains, forests, beaches, gardens, or flowing rivers, can be incredibly calming and restorative. Imagine the sights, sounds, smells, and sensations of being in nature, allowing yourself to fully immerse in the experience.

Body Scans: A body scan visualization involves systematically focusing your attention on different parts of your body, from your toes to the top of your head. This practice can help you develop greater body awareness, release tension, and promote deep relaxation.

Light Visualizations: Visualizing light, whether it's a warm golden light, a cool blue light (which can be particularly helpful when dealing with anger), a pure white light, or a vibrant rainbow of colors, can be a powerful way to promote healing, well-being, and spiritual connection. Imagine the light filling your body, clearing away any negativity, and leaving you feeling refreshed and revitalized.

Affirmations and Mantras: Combining visualization with positive affirmations or mantras can be a powerful way to reprogram your subconscious mind and cultivate positive beliefs about yourself. Visualize yourself embodying the qualities you desire, such as confidence, strength, or compassion, and repeat affirmations that reinforce these qualities. Mantras, whether they are faith-based prayers (like the Prayer of St. Francis) or sacred sounds (like "Om"), can also be incorporated into your visualizations, adding another layer of meaning and intention.

Personal Sanctuaries: Creating a visualization of a personal sanctuary, a place where you feel completely safe, comfortable, and at peace, can be a valuable tool for stress reduction and self-soothing. This sanctuary can be a real place you've visited or an imagined space that you create in your mind.

Spiritual Figures or Guides: If you have a spiritual practice or believe in a higher power, you can visualize connecting with spiritual figures or guides for inspiration, guidance, or support.

Creative Exploration: Allow your imagination to run free and explore any theme that resonates with you. You can visualize yourself achieving your goals, overcoming challenges, or simply exploring imaginative landscapes and scenarios.

VI. Chapter 6 Exercises:

Visualization Exercise 1: Your Peaceful Place

(A Creative Visualization)

Before you begin, please read through the entirety of Exercise 1 to familiarize yourself with the steps. Then, when you're ready, return to the beginning and follow the instructions at your own pace.

• **Getting Ready:** To enhance your visualization experience, consider adding a quiet background soundtrack. Nature sounds, soothing music, or ambient soundscapes can create a more immersive and relaxing atmosphere. If you choose to use sound, set up your sound source before you begin. Find a comfortable place where you can relax undisturbed for a few minutes. Close your eyes gently, or if that feels uncomfortable, simply soften your gaze. Take a few slow, deep breaths, allowing your body to settle and your mind to quiet.

• **Bring to mind a place that feels deeply peaceful,** soothing, and comforting to you. It could be a real place you've visited, a place you imagine, or a combination of both. Allow the image of this place to gently form in your mind's eye, spending a few minutes allowing this place to take shape while you explore your location getting sense of the scene before you.

• **What do you see in this place?** Notice the colors, the shapes, the light. Is it a wide-open landscape or a cozy, intimate space? Are there trees, water, a shoreline, mountains, or buildings? Allow your vision to become clear.

• **What do you hear in this place?** Are there sounds of nature, like birdsong or flowing water? Is there music, or is it quiet? Allow your ears to open to the sounds of your peaceful place, whether they are real or imagined.

• **What do you smell in this place?** Is there the scent of flowers, the fresh air after a rain, or the aroma of your favorite food? Allow your sense of smell to connect you to this place.

• **What do you feel in this place?** Is the air warm or cool on your skin? Are you sitting on soft grass or a comfortable chair? Allow your sense of touch to connect you to the physical sensations of your peaceful place.

• **What emotions do you feel in this place?** Do you feel calm, relaxed, joyful, content? Allow yourself to fully experience these positive emotions.

• **Take a few moments** to simply be in your peaceful place, savoring the sights, sounds, smells, sensations, and emotions. There's nothing to do here, nothing to achieve. Simply allow yourself to rest and recharge in this sanctuary of your own creation.

• **When you're ready,** gently bring your awareness back to your surroundings. Wiggle your fingers and toes, and when it feels right, slowly open your eyes. Carry the peace and comfort of your visualized place with you as you move through the rest of your day.

Visualization Exercise 2: Being the Mountain

(A Metaphorical Visualization)

Before you begin, please read through the entirety of Exercise 2 to familiarize yourself with the steps. Then, when you're ready, return to the beginning and follow the instructions at your own pace.

- **Getting Ready:** Find a comfortable place where you can relax undisturbed for a few minutes. You may wish to use a quiet background soundtrack of nature sounds or soothing music to enhance your experience. If so, set up your sound source before you begin. Close your eyes gently, or if that feels uncomfortable, simply soften your gaze. Take a few slow, deep breaths, allowing your body to settle and your mind to quiet.

- **Imagine yourself as a majestic mountain.** Feel the strength and stability in your base, rooted firmly in the earth. Your body is the mountain, solid and unmoving.

- **Visualize the sun rising and setting** on your mountain, the seasons changing around you. Feel the warmth of the summer sun on your slopes, the cool breeze of autumn rustling through your trees (if you have them). Imagine the snow falling gently on your peak in winter, and the vibrant green of spring as life returns to your slopes.

• **Feel the wind blowing against your face,** the rain washing over your surface. Imagine the snow piling up on your peak, the occasional lightning strike illuminating your form. These are the challenges of life, the ups and downs, the joys and sorrows, the triumphs and setbacks. The wind and rain shape your surface, but your essence remains strong and unyielding.

• **From the vantage point of your peak,** you have a panoramic unobstructed view of the landscape... the landscape of your life. You can easily see all the challenges, as well as the opportunities laid out before you, and you perceive them with natural clarity, insight, and wisdom.

• **Feel the solidity of your being,** the unwavering essence of your mountain self. You are a refuge, a place of peace and stability within.

• **Take a few moments to simply be the mountain,** feeling the strength and resilience that resides within you. There's nothing to do here, nothing to achieve. Simply allow yourself to rest in the unwavering fullness of your mountain self.

• **When you're ready,** gently bring your awareness back to your surroundings. Wiggle your fingers and toes, and when it feels right, slowly open your eyes. Carry the strength and resilience of your mountain self with you as you move through the rest of your day.

Visualization Conclusion:

So, dear reader, I hope you enjoyed these two visualization exercises. I invite you to explore the wide world of visualization, and all its variations if you feel inspired to do so, whether as a complement to your mindfulness efforts or simply as a delightful and restorative activity. Feel free to experiment with the exercises we've offered, and don't hesitate to explore the many resources for guided meditations and visualizations available through apps, audio-books, online resources, or in-person sessions. And who knows? Perhaps you'll be inspired to create your own visualizations, tailored to your unique needs and desires. The possibilities are as vast as your imagination. Enjoy the journey!

VII. Looking Ahead: Exploring Your Mindfulness Toolkit

Together we covered a lot in Chapter 6... but now we are ready to explore some real-world use cases to help prepare you for your continued journey with mindfulness. What you'll soon discover is that the tools you've already learned in this book can be applied to a wide range of life experiences and challenges.

The next set of chapters delve into specific areas where mindfulness can be particularly beneficial, offering practical strategies and insights for navigating life's ups and downs.

• **Chapter 7**, "Mindfulness for Emotional Well-being," explores how mindfulness techniques can support emotional regulation and resilience. It offers tools for managing everyday emotional challenges, provides strategies for de-escalating intense emotions, and emphasizes the importance of integrating mindfulness into daily life for sustained emotional well-being.

• **Chapter 8,** "Mindfulness for Pain and Discomfort," examines the complex nature of pain and how mindfulness can be a valuable complement to traditional pain management approaches. It introduces techniques like mindful breathing and body scans to help cultivate acceptance and reduce resistance to pain, emphasizing the importance of a holistic approach to well-being.

• **Chapter 9,** "Mindfulness for Grief, Loss, and Life Transitions," explores how mindfulness can support individuals through times of change and loss. It offers guidance on navigating grief, managing difficult emotions, and cultivating self-compassion and resilience during life transitions.

In these upcoming chapters I will introduce even more tools and additional insights that will expand and enhance your mindfulness toolkit, aiding your future journey toward greater ease, contentment, and clarity.

Conclusion for Chapter 6: Getting Ready for Life's Challenges

Congratulations! You've now explored a range of foundational mindfulness tools and techniques—from breath awareness and body scans to mindful movement, communication, and now, visualization—building a powerful foundation for your mindfulness journey.

Remember, this toolkit is yours. Personalize it, adjust it, and tweak it to align with your unique preferences and needs. There's no one-size-fits-all approach to mindfulness. Experiment, discover what resonates, and pay attention to what tools and approaches work best for you. The key is to use them! Familiarize yourself with these techniques so they're readily available when you need them, whether for daily support or to navigate life's larger challenges. And always check in with yourself to ensure these tools feel manageable, helpful, and supportive.

I hope the tools and insights in this chapter empower you to embrace life's journey with greater confidence, clarity, and ease. May your mindfulness adventures continue to deepen and enrich your life in countless ways.

Chapter 7

"Thoughts and emotions can be tumultuous.
Even one mindful breath can help."

Blair O'Neil (Author)

"You don't have to control your thoughts. You just
have to stop letting them control you."

Dan Millman

"We cannot prevent the birds of sorrow from
flying over our heads, but we can prevent them
from building nests in our hair."

Chinese Proverb

CHAPTER LEVEL TABLE OF CONTENTS

Chapter 7: Mindfulness for Emotional and Mental Well-being

Chapter 7

Mindfulness for Emotional and Mental Well-being

1. Introduction

Navigating our inner world of feelings and emotions can often feel like traversing a rocky and unpredictable path. While joy, contentment, and gratitude enrich our lives, challenging emotions can feel overwhelming and disruptive. This chapter focuses on managing the disruptive side of our emotions, as unchecked emotional upset can significantly impact our well-being and life satisfaction. My goal is to equip you with tools to navigate emotional upset and enjoy a greater sense mental and emotional equilibrium.

What You'll Find in This Chapter

In this chapter, I'll explore several practical ways to use mindfulness to navigate our emotional and mental turbulence and support our emotional stability and resilience. While mindfulness isn't a magic cure, it does provide an effective framework for managing life's upsets and supporting our calm even amidst the challenges. **There are times when emotions are so intense and overwhelming—what we might call "emotional storms"—that traditional mindfulness practices are difficult to implement.** To address these intense experiences, we've included a dedicated section offering immediate, action-oriented strategies for managing such moments later in this chapter *(see pages 173 to 178)*.

Not a Substitute for Professional Support:

It's important to note that the information in this book is not intended as a substitute for professional medical or mental health advice. If you are experiencing significant physical, emotional or mental health challenges, please seek the guidance of a qualified healthcare professional.

II. Understanding Emotional and Mental Challenges

First, together we'll explore the milder emotions in the A and B sections that follow. Here is a brief explanation of how I are presenting the two aspects of emotions:

• **Section A. The emotions that are primarily physiological in nature** (Stress, Anxiety, and Worry),

• **Section B. The emotions that are primarily emotional and cognitive** (Anger, Sadness, Fear, Grief, Shame, and Guilt).

Following these two sections, then I will explore the more upsetting "emotional storms," where traditional mindfulness techniques may not be sufficient, and provide several immediate action steps, strategies and resources to help you navigate those emotional storms.

Our Inner Emotional Landscape: Mild to Moderate Upsets

Section A. Worry, Anxiety, and Stress

Worry, anxiety, and stress are common experiences in our modern world. While some stress can be a normal part of life and even a helpful motivator at times, excessive or chronic worry, anxiety, and stress can significantly and negatively impact both our physical and mental well-being. This section explores the specifics of how mindfulness helps us navigate life's inevitable stressors and upsets.

What It Feels Like (Subjective Experiences): Like other difficult emotions, worry, anxiety, and stress can create a wide range of internal experiences that can be both uncomfortable and confusing.

- **Worry often feels like a mental hamster wheel,** with thoughts endlessly circling around potential problems or negative outcomes. It's like your mind is stuck on repeat, replaying "what if" scenarios and rehearsing worst-case possibilities. It can feel like a constant mental chatter that you just can't seem to stop, making it difficult to focus on the present moment.

- **Anxiety can feel different;** it might show up as a knot in your stomach, a sense of unease or dread, or a feeling of being constantly on edge, like waiting for the other shoe to drop. You might experience racing thoughts, difficulty concentrating, and a sense of being overwhelmed. At its most intense, anxiety can manifest as an anxiety attack, which can involve a sudden surge of intense fear or panic, accompanied by physical symptoms like rapid heart rate, shortness of breath, chest pain, dizziness, and trembling. It can feel like you're losing control or even having a heart attack.

• **Stress, on the other hand,** can feel like a heavy weight on your shoulders, a sense of being overwhelmed or pressured, or a feeling of being constantly pulled in different directions. It can manifest as irritability, difficulty sleeping, and a sense of being constantly "on," as if you're running on empty, struggling to keep up with the demands of daily life. It's important to remember that these experiences, while often intertwined, are distinct and can show up in different ways for different people.

How It Shows Up (Objective/Physical Symptoms):
Worry, anxiety, and stress, while they are often experienced mentally and emotionally, they also have distinct ways of showing up in our bodies in ways that can be quite challenging to manage.

These physical signs and body sensations can vary in intensity and duration, so it's important to remember that they may also overlap leading to some degree of confusion about what you are feeling.

The important thing is to learn to recognize them, which in turn then becomes a valuable tool for understanding your emotional state and how best to face and work with those emotional challenges:

• **Worry:** While worry is primarily a mental process, it can still manifest physically. Some common physical signs include: difficulty sleeping (especially trouble falling asleep or staying asleep), muscle tension (particularly in the jaw, neck, and shoulders), headaches, and stomach upset.

• **Anxiety:** Anxiety often has a more pronounced physical component. Common physical signs of anxiety include: rapid heartbeat or palpitations, shortness of breath or hyperventilation, chest pain or tightness, dizziness or lightheadedness, sweating, trembling or shaking, muscle tension, stomach upset or nausea, and feeling restless or on edge. As mentioned earlier, at its most intense, anxiety can manifest as an anxiety attack, which involves a sudden surge of these symptoms.

• **Stress:** Stress can manifest in a wide range of physical ways, including: headaches, muscle tension (especially in the neck, shoulders, and back), fatigue, difficulty sleeping, changes in appetite (either loss of appetite or overeating), stomach upset or digestive problems, and a weakened immune system (leading to more frequent colds or illnesses).

Section B. Anger, Sadness, Fear, Grief, Shame, and Guilt

Emotions like anger, sadness, fear, grief, shame, and guilt are also a natural part of the human experience. However, these emotions can be experienced differently than the worry, anxiety, and stress we just described in **Section A**.

This new set of emotions can often feel weightier, more oppressive, and more complex than our normal everyday stress or anxiety. These emotions can stir up deep-seated fears or challenge long-held foundational beliefs, and even trigger past traumas, bringing them forward into the current moment, while also negatively impacting our sense of self.

Later in this section, we will explore how mindfulness can offer valuable tools for working with these challenging emotions, fostering greater self-compassion, acceptance, and a fuller understanding of our inner emotional world.

What It Feels Like (Subjective Experiences): And like the emotions we discussed of anxiety, stress, and worry, other difficult emotions can manifest in a wide variety of ways, creating a range of internal experiences that can be as uncomfortable as they are confusing.

You might feel overwhelmed by a wave of intense feeling, or you might experience a more subtle, persistent unease. Sometimes these emotions can feel like they're taking over, making it hard to think clearly or act rationally. Other times, you might feel numb or disconnected, as if you're watching your life from a distance.

It's important to remember that all emotions are valid and a natural part of the human experience. Here are some examples of how specific emotions might feel:

- **Anger:** Can feel like heat rising in your body, a tightening in your chest or jaw, or an urge to lash out. It can feel like an internal pressure cooker, ready to explode.

- **Sadness:** Can feel like a heaviness in your chest, a sense of emptiness or hollowness, or a desire to withdraw from the world. It's like a gray cloud has settled over your mind, making it hard to see the light.

- **Fear:** Can feel like a racing heart, shallow breathing, or a sense of panic. It's like being frozen in place, unable to move or think.

- **Grief:** Can feel like a deep ache in your heart, a sense of disbelief or numbness, or waves of intense sadness that come and go. It's like a piece of you is missing, leaving a profound sense of loss.

- **Shame:** Can feel like a burning embarrassment, a desire to hide or disappear. It's like a spotlight is shining on your perceived flaws, making you feel exposed and vulnerable.

• **Guilt:** Can feel like a heavy weight on your conscience, a sense of remorse or regret. It's like you're constantly replaying a past mistake, judging yourself harshly.

How It Shows Up (Objective/Physical Symptoms):
Difficult emotions, usually experienced as something "inside of us," very often show up in our bodies in lots of different ways, from simple sensations to more obvious outward expressions.

The degree and intensity of these physical signs can vary dramatically, depending on the specific emotion or combination of emotions being experienced. Recognizing these physical signs is a valuable tool for becoming more aware of your emotional state and lessening their negative impact.

It's important to remember that many of these physical signs can and often do overlap. For example, muscle tension can be associated with anger, fear, and guilt. These emotions, whether experienced individually or in combination, can trigger the body's stress responses.

Understanding these outward expressions and recognizing the potential for overlapping physical sensations can help us better understand our emotional experiences. It's also important to realize that these physical experiences can sometimes be so strong or severe that they are mistaken for physical illnesses.

This highlights the vital connection between our emotional and physical well-being and how this awareness can help us navigate our emotional landscape.

Here are some examples of how different emotions might show up in body:

- **Anger:** Clenched fists or jaw, flushed face, rapid breathing, increased heart rate, muscle tension (especially in the shoulders and neck).

- **Sadness:** Slumped posture, tearfulness, heavy limbs, fatigue, loss of appetite or overeating.

- **Fear:** Rapid heartbeat, shallow breathing, sweating, trembling, muscle tension, butterflies in the stomach.

- **Grief:** Tightness in the chest, shortness of breath, fatigue, changes in sleep patterns, loss of appetite.

- **Shame:** Blushing, feeling hot or flushed, sinking feeling in the stomach, wanting to hide or disappear.

- **Guilt:** Tightness in the chest, stomach aches, feeling restless or agitated, difficulty sleeping.

Mindfulness in Daily Life: Cultivating Emotional Stability & Strength

First, let's put mindfulness into a larger context of "when and how to use it". We have to remember that mindfulness isn't just something you "do" during formal meditation sessions or a scheduled "practice time" (if you engage in such formal approaches); I think it's best viewed as a life-enhancing tool, accessible in almost any situation, regardless of your experience level. In the case of emotional support, mindfulness offers three key benefits:

1. The ability to cultivate greater emotional resilience (not be derailed by emotional upsets)

2. The ability to cultivate greater emotional stability (calmer when facing emotional challenges)

3. Faster recovery from emotional upsets

By bringing mindful awareness into our everyday activities, we can not only meet our everyday emotional challenges with greater ease, but also create a strong foundation for navigating any future emotional upsets and upheavals.

Practical Tips & Strategies

Here are some practical ways to use mindfulness in your daily life to cultivate emotional resilience:

• **Mindful Moments:** Throughout the day, take short "mindful moments" to notice what emotions are present. Pause for a few breaths and notice what emotions are present (from ease and contentment to low-grade stress and beyond). Notice what sensations you're experiencing in your body and what thoughts are arising in response to your emotions.

◇ These mindful moments can help you identify early warning signs of escalating emotions and take proactive steps to prevent them from becoming overwhelming.

• **Mindful Activities:** When bringing mindful awareness to everyday activities, such as brushing your teeth, washing dishes, or walking, you can also perform an "emotion scan" to see if your emotions are active and influencing these activities. For example, if you're feeling frustrated while washing dishes, you might notice yourself scrubbing harder, having harsh thoughts, or engaging in negative self-talk. Use these moments as opportunities to work with the RAIN technique with the arising or fully felt emotion *(see page 172).*

◊ This technique can help you develop greater awareness of how emotions manifest in your daily life and build your capacity to respond to them with greater skill.

• **Mindful Transitions:** Use transitions between activities as opportunities to check in with your emotions (both pleasant and challenging). For example, before getting out of your car after a stressful commute, take a moment to notice your breath and how you're feeling. Or, before starting a new task at work after a difficult conversation, take a few seconds to center yourself and acknowledge any lingering emotions.

◊ These short pauses can help you avoid carrying emotions from one activity to the next and create space for a fresh start.

• **Mindfulness After an Emotional Storm:** After experiencing an emotional storm *(see pages 173 to 178)* and utilizing the immediate strategies we discussed, returning to mindfulness techniques can be particularly beneficial.

◇ Using techniques like Recognizing and Accepting Emotions, Observing Sensations, Working with Thoughts, and RAIN can help you process the experience, gain insights into the triggers and patterns involved, and prevent similar escalations in the future. This is a crucial step in building long-term emotional resilience. *(see page 172 for RAIN information.)*

Examples and Success Stories:

• **Example 1:** Managing Worry and Anxiety: Robert *(name changed)* found himself constantly worrying about his health and finances, especially after retiring. His worries kept him up at night and made it difficult to enjoy his days. He began practicing mindful breathing exercises, focusing on the sensation of his breath entering and leaving his body. He learned to recognize when his mind wandered to worries and gently redirect his attention back to his breath. By practicing regularly, Robert noticed a significant reduction in his anxiety. He also found it easier to be present in the moment and to shift his worrying into actionable steps to improve his financial situation and address his concerns, including budgeting and researching resources for financial planning. This became easier as he learned to recognize that his worries were just thoughts, not necessarily facts.

• **Example 2:** Working with Grief and Sadness: Similarly, after the loss of a close friend, Eleanor *(name changed)* experienced deep sadness and grief. She felt overwhelmed by waves of emotion and struggled to find any joy in her usual activities. Recognizing the intensity of her grief, she also sought support from a grief support group in addition to starting to work with the RAIN technique, as described earlier in this chapter, recognizing her sadness, allowing it to be present without resistance, investigating the physical sensations associated with it (a heavy feeling in her chest), and reminding herself that she was not defined by her grief. The RAIN technique, along with the support from her grief group, helped Eleanor to process her grief in a more accepting and compassionate way.

• **Example 3:** Dealing with Anger and Frustration: Another individual, George *(name changed)*, often felt irritable and easily frustrated, especially when dealing with technology or changes in his routine. He began practicing mindful awareness of his emotions, noticing the physical sensations of anger rising in his body (clenched fists, rapid heartbeat). By observing these sensations without judgment, he was able to create a small space between the feeling of anger and his reaction to it. This allowed him to choose a more thoughtful response which gave rise to feelings of patience and calm.

• **Example 4:** Integrating Mindfulness into Daily Life: Finally, consider this example of Helen *(name changed)* who was initially skeptical about mindfulness but decided to try incorporating mindful moments into her daily routine. She started by bringing awareness to simple activities like drinking her morning coffee, noticing the taste, smell, and warmth of the cup in her hands. She also began practicing mindful walking, paying attention to the sensation of her feet on the ground. Through these simple exercises, Helen found that she felt more grounded and present throughout her day, even during stressful situations. She also began to notice a newfound appreciation for the everyday moments and experiences she had grown accustomed to and was no longer interacting with in meaningful ways.

III. Techniques & Strategies for Managing Emotional Upsets:

Mindfulness Techniques for Mild to Moderate Emotional Challenges

Now that we've explored these emotional experiences, let's turn to practical ways mindfulness can help us navigate everyday emotional upsets.

What About Extreme Emotional Upset?

For more severe, overwhelming, or debilitating emotional experiences, please refer to the following section on pages 173 to 178 titled "Mindfulness & Emotional Storms: Immediate Strategies for Intense Emotions."

Using the Tools of Mindfulness:

Think of the following mindfulness techniques as tools in a toolbox. You wouldn't necessarily use every tool in the box for every task. Similarly, you can choose to use one, two, three, or all of these mindfulness tools, depending on your needs and preferences. You may find that one technique resonates more with you than others, or you may choose to combine several techniques depending on the situation.

The key is to experiment and find what works best for you.

In this section, we will explore the five key Mindfulness Tools:

1. *Recognizing and Accepting Emotions*

2. *Observing Sensations*

3. *Working with Thoughts*

4. *The RAIN Technique (A commonly used approach)*

5. *The Heart of Mindfulness—Being Present Now*

Mindfulness Tool Option 1: Recognizing and Accepting Emotions

• **Becoming aware of your emotions** as they arise, without bias, agenda, judgment or suppression

• **Acknowledging that emotions** are a natural part of the human experience

• **Allowing yourself to feel your emotions** fully, without trying to resist or push them away. (This acceptance is key to working with emotions mindfully.)

Mindfulness Tool Option 2: Observing Sensations

• Bringing mindful awareness to the physical sensations associated with your emotions.

• Noticing how your body feels when you're experiencing stress, anxiety, or other emotions

• Observing sensations such as tightness in the chest, rapid heartbeat, or tension in the shoulders.

• You can also apply a similar approach to exploring your emotions. Try to "find" the emotion in your body. Where do you feel it? What are the specific sensations?

◇ *For example, if you're feeling anxious,* you might notice a tightness in your chest or a fluttering in your stomach. Try to locate the edges of this sensation. Does it feel like a knot, a flutter, or a pressure? Is the sensation the same throughout the area, or are there variations in intensity? What is the quality of the sensation—is it sharp, dull, throbbing, or constant? What is the texture of the sensation? Does it feel hot or cold, tight or loose? What is the size of the sensation? Does it stay in one place or does it move around? What thoughts or images arise when you focus on the sensation? How does the breath change when you bring awareness to the sensation?

◊ *If you're feeling sad,* you might notice a heaviness in your chest or a lump in your throat. Again, try to explore the qualities of this sensation in detail. Where does the sadness seem to live in your body? What are the edges of the feeling? What does it feel like where the sadness meets the rest of your body? What are the thoughts and images that arise when you focus on the sadness?

The key is to observe the sensations with a gentle spirit of curiosity and self-inquiry, without bias, agenda or judgment, just as you would in the "Find the Pain" exercise.

Mindfulness Tool Option 3: Working with Thoughts

- **Becoming aware of the thoughts** that accompany your emotions

- **Recognize thoughts as thoughts, not facts**

- **Gently guiding your attention** away from negative or unhelpful thought patterns

Mindfulness Tool Option 4: The RAIN Technique

- **Recognize:** Gently acknowledge and be softly aware of any emotions that are present

- **Allow:** Allow the emotion without suppression, resistance, bias, or any agenda

- **Investigate:** Gently observe the emotion with curiosity in the spirit of inquiry. Notice where you feel it in your body, the thoughts that accompany it, and any physical sensations

- **Non-identification:** Remember that you are not your emotions. You are the awareness that is observing the emotion

Mindfulness Tool Option 5: The Heart of Mindfulness—Being Present Now

This is the foundation of all mindfulness awareness. It is the very essence of mindfulness—simply being present with whatever is arising in this very moment, without bias, judgment, striving, or agenda. There is no goal to achieve, nothing to fix or change. It is simply being here, now, with the ungraspable, yet apparent, fully experienced, kaleidoscopic moment of now. It is from this place of awareness that all other mindfulness techniques arise.

X. Mindfulness & Emotional Storms: Immediate Strategies for Intense Emotions

During intense 'emotional storms' or 'emotional tornadoes,' traditional mindfulness techniques may be difficult or impossible to implement. These moments require immediate, action-oriented strategies including to help sooth and calm your reactions. The following tips, tools, and techniques are can be helpful during emotional storms:

- **Remove yourself from the emotional trigger:** This is often the most crucial first step. Physically removing yourself from the source of the emotional distress creates the space you need to begin to regulate your emotions. This might involve:

   ◊ *Going outside for a walk* or simply stepping away from the immediate situation.

   ◊ *Moving to another room* where you can close the door and have some privacy.

   ◊ *Asking the person* (or people) involved in the situation to give you some space.

- **Shift Your Mental & Sensory Focus** (without specific mindfulness techniques): A simple and powerful way to shift your upset is to intentionally engage in your immediate surroundings. This might be as simple as counting the books on a shelf, naming all the blue things you can see, or counting fence posts or cars as they pass by. This technique gives your mind a simple and effective way to reset and calm your upset. *(For more on this DBT-inspired technique, please see Appendix A, Page 347)*

• **Move your body** (without specific mindfulness techniques): Physical movement can be a powerful way to release pent-up emotional energy and begin to regulate your nervous system. This isn't about "mindful movement" in the traditional sense, where you focus on the sensations of the body or count your steps. In this context, the goal is to use physical activity to shift your emotional state and dissipate intense emotional energy. Some effective strategies include:

◊ *Walking, running, or cycling outdoors,* preferably in nature and away from crowds if possible. (These are particularly beneficial for seniors, as they are generally accessible and provide a good balance of physical activity and connection with nature.)

◊ *Pacing in a room or hallway.*

◊ *Engaging in other forms of physical activity,* such as stretching, yoga, or even simple movements like rubbing your arms, legs, or face.

◊ *Engaging larger muscle groups* through activities like "wall pushing" or squeezing and releasing pillows or tension balls (bigger is better, in many cases).

◊ *For some, "getting squeezed"* (through hugs, weighted blankets, or even wearing a heavy coat) can also provide a sense of comfort and calm.

• **Engage your breath** (without specific mindfulness techniques). This simple act can provide a powerful anchor in the midst of emotional turmoil. Important Considerations:

◊ *In the midst of an emotional storm,* complex mindfulness breathing techniques might be difficult to implement. Instead, focus on simple, conscious deep breaths.

◊ *This isn't about "mindful breathing"* per se (counting breaths or focusing on the sensation of the breath); it's simply about taking deep, conscious breaths to help dissipate the intense emotional energy.

• **Do No Harm:** This is a crucial principle during intense emotional states: avoid any actions that could harm yourself, others, or property. This includes:

• **Avoiding verbal outbursts:** Don't yell at others, try to explain yourself in a highly emotional state, threaten anyone, or lash out with hurtful words.

• **Avoiding dangerous activities:** Don't drive a motor vehicle, operate machinery, or engage in any activity that requires focus and clear judgment.

• **Avoid accessing firearms:** During periods of intense emotional distress, it is absolutely crucial to avoid accessing firearms. Even if you don't have immediate thoughts of self-harm or harming others, the presence of a firearm can significantly increase the risk of impulsive and potentially irreversible actions. If you have firearms in your home, ensure they are securely stored and inaccessible during these times. If you are concerned about your safety or the safety of others, consider temporarily removing firearms from the home.

• **Avoid misusing medications** (prescription or over-the-counter), alcohol, or other substances during emotional distress: This is particularly important for seniors, as many may have access to a variety of prescription medications and may be more susceptible to the effects of alcohol and other substances. During emotional distress, the temptation to use these substances to numb or escape feelings can be strong

⋄ *Misusing any of these substances* can be extremely dangerous, leading to accidental overdose, adverse drug interactions, worsening of underlying emotional problems, or other health complications.

⋄ *If you are feeling overwhelmed,* please reach out for professional support instead of turning to substances.

• **Avoiding other self-destructive behaviors:** Don't throw or break things, and don't physically hurt yourself or others.

- **Reset and Seek Support:** The goal of these immediate strategies is to reset your emotional state and bring down before resuming normal activities.

  ◇ *This might mean taking a break for several hours,* a day, or even longer, depending on the intensity of the emotional experience.

  ◇ *Only when you feel truly capable of engaging without being overwhelmed* or reactive should you return to triggering environments or interactions.

  ◇ *Once the intensity of the emotional storm has subsided,* you may find it helpful to revisit the mindfulness techniques described earlier in this chapter (Recognizing and Accepting Emotions, Observing Sensations, Working with Thoughts, and RAIN) to further process the experience and prevent future emotional escalations.

  ◇ *Continue using self-soothing measures as needed.*

- **For immediate danger to yourself or others, call 911** (or your local emergency number): If you are experiencing thoughts of harming yourself or others, or if you feel you are losing control and may act in a way that could cause harm, it is crucial to seek immediate help. Calling 911 (or your local emergency number) can connect you to emergency services who can provide immediate assistance.

• **For non-emergency support:** It's also important to access other support services as appropriate and available. These might include:

  ◇ 988 Suicide & Crisis Lifeline (in the United States)

  ◇ 12-Step Support Groups

  ◇ Church or faith-based groups

  ◇ Issue-specific peer support groups (for anger management, grief, cancer, abuse, etc.)

  ◇ Veterans support groups

  ◇ PTSD support groups

  ◇ Survivor groups

  ◇ Mental health professionals

V. Conclusion: Integrating Mindfulness and Seeking Support

Mindfulness is a valuable tool for navigating the full range of our emotional experiences, from everyday stress to more intense emotional challenges we all face from time to time.

However, it's important to recognize that mindfulness is not a substitute for professional mental health care.

If you are experiencing intense or prolonged emotional distress that significantly impacts your daily life, relationships, or work; if you find yourself struggling to manage your emotions even with consistent mindfulness practice; if you experience persistent physical symptoms related to emotional distress; or, most importantly, if you are having thoughts of self-harm or suicide, please seek immediate help from a qualified mental health professional or by contacting emergency services.

Seeking help is a sign of strength, not weakness, and a courageous step toward healing and well-being.

VI. Looking Ahead to Chapter 8: Mindfulness for Pain & Discomfort

Having explored mindfulness for emotional well-being, next we'll now turn our attention to another area where mindful awareness can be profoundly helpful: physical pain. The following chapter examines how these same principles can be applied to manage physical sensations, reduce suffering, and cultivate greater resilience in the face of pain and discomfort.

Chapter 8

"Pain is inevitable. Suffering is optional."

Haruki Murakami

"The wound is the place
where the Light enters you."

Rumi

"Pain cannot be ignored or wished away.
But underneath the clanging noise of the pain there
is a deep wholeness that can be re-inhabited if,
just for a moment, we could approach willingly..."

Mark Williams

CHAPTER LEVEL TABLE OF CONTENTS

Chapter 8: Mindfulness for Pain & Discomfort

Chapter 8

Mindfulness for Pain & Discomfort

Long Chapter Ahead:

There are a lot of information to present when discussing Pain & Discomfort topics. I have endeavored to keep the explanations as simple as possible while also trying to relay both relevant and helpful information. Take your time with this chapter as there is a lot to consider and absorb.

I. Navigating the Pain & Discomfort Landscape

We all have a unique and evolving relationship with pain and discomfort. For some, the body's journey is relatively gentle. For others, it's marked by injuries, chronic conditions, or the natural changes of aging. Regardless of our experiences, most of us eventually reach a point—often in our senior years—where our bodies don't function or heal as they once did.

How we relate to these universal experiences of pain—from occasional reminders to persistent signals, and whether we react with acceptance, denial, or avoidance—shapes our experience of pain.

This chapter focuses on our relationship with pain and discomfort and its impact on our daily lives, emotional well-being, and overall quality of life. From a nagging headache to the ongoing reality of chronic pain, these sensations can be a constant companion and a significant challenge, especially for seniors. Here, we begin our journey to understanding and working with pain and discomfort through the techniques of mindfulness.

Understanding the Scope of Pain and Discomfort

While pain and discomfort are universal, our experiences and perceptions of them are deeply personal and varied. What one person perceives as a minor ache, another might experience as debilitating pain.

It's important to remember that our experience of pain is unique, it is not only a physical sensation; it has far-reaching effects—what we might call the 'tentacles of pain'—that profoundly impact our emotions, thoughts, behaviors, often leading to feelings of frustration, anger, anxiety, sadness, and even desperation.

In short, it can be a major life-disruptor, affecting our sleep, daily activities, relationships, and our enjoyment of life. In this chapter, we will explore this multifaceted nature of pain and discomfort, and its physical, emotional, and mental dimensions. We will also introduce mindfulness approaches to help navigating these challenges with greater calm, and intention.

Mindfulness: A Whole-Person Complementary Approach

While mindfulness offers an effective and flexible framework for navigating the challenging landscape of pain and discomfort, **it's important to emphasize that mindfulness is not a cure for pain, nor is it a replacement for medical care.**

Rather, mindfulness is best thought of as a complementary approach or life tool that can be used either on its own or in conjunction with other traditional therapeutics or alternative health approaches.

The key point is that mindfulness helps us change our relationship with pain. By cultivating a mindful approach, we can learn to experience pain with less reactivity, resistance and upheaval.

By reducing our unintended but understandable struggles with pain—the emotional reactivity, anger, blame, victim hood—we can begin to shift our experience of pain.

Important Note:

While mindfulness can be a helpful tool for many, it's important to acknowledge that focusing on pain can be challenging or even distressing for some individuals, particularly those with severe or chronic pain.

If you find any of this information or the following exercises to be overwhelming, upsetting, or triggering, please stop. Consider consulting with your healthcare provider or a qualified mental health professional if needed.

What You'll Find in This Chapter:

In this chapter, we will explore practical mindfulness techniques, including present moment awareness, that can help you:

- Understand the different types and experiences of pain and discomfort.

- Manage the emotional distress associated with pain.

- Cultivate greater acceptance of pain and reduce resistance, helping you change your relationship with pain.

- Integrate mindfulness with other supportive approaches.

- Adapt mindfulness techniques to different contexts and situations.

I will also touch on when to seek professional medical support for assistance with your pain management, and emphasize that seeking support is a sign of strength, not weakness.

II. Understanding Pain and Discomfort

Before exploring how mindfulness can help us navigate personal experiences of pain and discomfort, it's essential to establish a basic understanding of the different types of pain and how they can change over time. This foundational knowledge will inform both our coping and management strategies and enhance the effectiveness of the mindfulness techniques we'll explore. Let's set the stage.

Defining Pain and Discomfort:

Let's take a moment to clarify the definitions of pain and discomfort. This is an important distinction to understand as we explore these sensations, our relationship to them, and how mindfulness can play a positive role.

Pain and discomfort, while often used interchangeably, are actually distinct experiences.

Pain is generally defined as an unpleasant sensory and emotional experience associated with actual or potential tissue damage. Think of it as a complex interplay of physical, emotional, and mental components—a truly multifaceted experience. **Discomfort,** on the other hand, is usually a milder sensation. It can range from a slight ache or stiffness to a feeling of unease. While it doesn't always mean tissue damage, it can sometimes signal a potential for injury. **And just like pain, discomfort also has an emotional component.** This can range from mild annoyance or impatience to frustration or even anxiety, especially when discomfort is persistent or chronic. **Discomfort can sometimes be a precursor to pain,** a lingering sensation after pain has subsided, or simply a mild annoyance.

Types of Pain:

Pain can manifest in diverse ways, depending on its cause, duration, and individual experience. Let's explore the two main categories: acute and chronic pain.

• **Acute pain is typically short-lived,** lasting from a few minutes to a few months (sometimes up to six months). Think of it as a warning signal from your body, arising from a specific injury, surgery, or illness. It usually has a clear cause and resolves as the underlying issue heals. The intensity of acute pain can range from mild to severe.

• **Chronic pain is defined as pain that persists for longer than three months** or past the normal healing time for the initial injury or cause. This can be due to ongoing conditions like arthritis, nerve damage (neuropathic pain), fibromyalgia, or other chronic illnesses. **It's also important to recognize that some injuries, especially in older adults, may be slow**

to heal or may not heal completely due to factors like circulatory issues, age-related changes in the skin, or long-term medication use (such as steroids). This can lead to persistent or chronic pain even if the initial injury wasn't severe. Chronic pain can significantly impact a person's physical and emotional well-being and often requires a multidisciplinary approach to management.

While acute and chronic pain are the primary classifications, pain can also be categorized based on its origin. These categories—while often considered subcategories of acute or chronic pain—represent very real experiences for those living with them. Understanding the spectrum of pain types can be helpful in navigating your own pain journey. Here are some examples:

- **Injury-related pain:** This can be either acute (e.g., ranging from major trauma to a sprained ankle) or chronic (e.g., ongoing back pain).

- **Post-surgical pain:** This is typically acute in the immediate aftermath of surgery, but it can sometimes become chronic.

- **Illness-related pain:** This can also be acute (e.g., pain from an infection) or chronic (e.g., pain from arthritis).

The Cyclical Nature of Pain:

Though it may feel like it, pain is rarely a static experience. It often follows a cyclical, wavelike pattern, with periods of increasing intensity (progression), easing of pain (regression), varying levels of pain (fluctuations), and periods of much worse pain (flare-ups). Understanding these pain cycles can help us better accept what is happening and manage our pain experiences.

III. Pain in Our Lives

General Considerations When Experiencing Pain:
Before exploring how pain can manifest in different contexts and areas of our lives, let's consider some general principles that apply to all pain experiences:

• **The Unique Nature of Pain:** Each person's experience of pain is unique, influenced by factors such as the type and intensity of pain, personal history, coping mechanisms, and emotional state.

• **The Impact of Approach:** How we approach pain—whether with resistance, acceptance, rushing, or mindful awareness—can significantly influence our experience.

• **The Interplay of Physical, Emotional, and Mental Factors:** Pain is a complex experience involving physical sensations, emotional responses, and mental processes.

- **The Importance of Self-Care and Self-Kindness:**
It's important to approach pain with kindness and understanding towards ourselves.

Pain at Home:

Home is often considered a sanctuary, a place of comfort and refuge. Yet, for many of us, it can also become a primary location where pain is experienced, sometimes even most acutely. Whether it's the familiar stiffness of arthritis in the morning, a nagging backache after household chores, the lingering effects of an old injury flaring up, or the constant experience of chronic pain, these sensations can disrupt our daily routines and diminish our enjoyment of our personal space. The very place where we seek comfort can become a source of frustration and distress.

Pain at the Doctor's Office/Urgent Care/Emergency Room:

Visiting a doctor's office, urgent care, or emergency room can be a source of stress and anxiety for many of us, even when we're not dealing with pain. When pain is part of the picture—whether it's acute pain from a recent injury or illness, the ongoing challenge of chronic pain, or even just a follow-up appointment to discuss past pain—those feelings of stress and anxiety can become much stronger.

The clinical environment itself—with its unfamiliar sights, sounds, and procedures—can heighten our sensitivity to pain and make us feel more vulnerable. Waiting for appointments, undergoing examinations, interacting with staff we don't know, and discussing potentially concerning diagnoses can all contribute to increased tension and discomfort.

Pain During a Hospital Stay:

A hospital stay, even for a planned procedure, can be a disorienting and stressful experience. Being in an unfamiliar environment, surrounded by medical equipment and unfamiliar routines, can heighten our awareness of physical sensations, including pain. The constant interruptions for tests, medications, and nurse or doctor assessments can further disrupt sleep and create a sense of unease, making pain feel even more pronounced.

Pain During Daily Activities:

For many people living with pain, everyday tasks and activities can become significant challenges. From simple chores like grocery shopping, getting the mail, or doing laundry, to more involved activities like work, hobbies, or social engagements, pain can disrupt our routines and limit our ability to participate fully in life. Even activities we once enjoyed can become sources of frustration and discomfort.

Unique Experiences For Everyone

It's essential to understand that everyone experiences pain differently. What might be a minor twinge for one person could be debilitating for another. This isn't a matter of weakness or strength; it's a reflection of the complex interplay of various factors that influence our individual pain perception. These factors include:

- **The type of pain:** Is it sharp, dull, burning, throbbing, or aching? Different types of pain can have different causes and require different approaches.

- **The intensity of the pain:** How severe is the pain on a scale of 0 to 10? Even the same type of pain can be experienced at vastly different intensities.

- **Our personal history with pain:** Have we experienced similar pain before? Past experiences can shape our expectations and reactions to current pain.

- **Our overall physical health:** Existing health conditions, such as diabetes or arthritis, or current or past injuries, can affect pain perception and healing.

- **Our emotional and mental state:** Stress, anxiety, depression, and other emotional factors can significantly influence how we perceive and cope with pain.

- **Our coping mechanisms and support systems:** How do we typically deal with difficult situations? Do we have a strong support network of family, friends, or healthcare providers?

- **Our cultural background and beliefs:** Cultural norms and beliefs about pain can influence how we express and manage it.

- **Our living situation and daily demands:**
Our living environment, work demands, and family responsibilities can all affect how pain impacts our lives.

These factors interact in complex ways, layering and affecting each other, creating a unique pain experience for each individual. It's important to remember that there is no "right" or "wrong" way to experience pain. Your pain is uniquely yours and absolutely a legitimate experience at whatever level you experience it. It's essential to approach it with gentleness, understanding, as much self-care and support as you need.

Your Approach Can Affect Things:

As individuals, how we approach pain—whether with resistance, acceptance, rushing, or avoidance—can significantly influence our experience of the pain. When we resist pain, we often tense our muscles, hold our breath, and engage in negative self-talk. This can actually amplify the pain and create a cycle of suffering.

For example, if we're experiencing a backache or neck ache while doing chores, and we try to push through it without acknowledging the discomfort or adjusting our movements, we're likely to make the pain worse. Similarly, becoming overwhelmed by anxiety or fear when experiencing severe pain can heighten our sensitivity and make it more difficult to cope.

The Mindfulness Role

Simply said, mindfulness offers a valuable tool in the arsenal of living with pain. By bringing a mindful approach to the experience, we can begin to witness pain sensations, but without critical self-talk, dramatic over-elaboration of our "pain story," or taking on habitual roles (eg, victim, hero, etc), and in many cases, reduce the intensity of our pain perceptions. This doesn't mean we have to like the pain or discomfort, or avoid taking action to address the source of the pain through medical interventions or other support systems. In short, by using the approach of pain-awareness, we are able to create a space or buffer between the sensations of pain and our reaction to them. This allows us to make more conscious and calmer choices about how to respond, such as modifying our activities, taking a break, working with relaxation techniques, or using other pain management strategies. A common additional benefit of a mindful journey with pain, it tends to give rise to the compassionate understanding that pain, in whatever form it takes, is a common human experience and that we are not alone in our suffering.

The Impact of Pain on Relationships:

Let's face it, pain doesn't exist in a vacuum. It's not just a physical sensation; it ripples outwards, affecting every aspect of our lives – from how we move and what we can do, to how we connect with the world around us. And perhaps one of the most significant impacts is on our relationships—those vital connections with family, friends, caregivers, and even casual acquaintances. This is a topic close to all of our hearts, because our relationships are so fundamental to our sense of self and our overall well-being. So, let's explore how pain can play a powerful role in shaping these important connections.

- **Pain and Our Relationships:** Living with pain doesn't just affect us physically and emotionally; as we said, it can also ripple outwards, impacting our the people in our lives. It's tough when pain becomes a constant companion because it can change our relationship dynamics and how we interact with others—family members (including spouses, children, siblings, and parents), close friends, caregivers (including medical professionals and home health aides), and even acquaintances and members of our community—often in ways we don't even realize.

- **The Spectrum of Pain and Its Emotional Impact:** It's important to recognize that pain manifests in many ways, and these different types of pain can have unique effects on our relationships. Acute pain, like that from a recent injury, might lead to temporary limitations and a need for increased support. Chronic pain, on the other hand, can create ongoing challenges and require long-term adjustments in roles and responsibilities. Regardless of the type of pain, the emotional and mental toll—including frustration, irritability, anxiety, and even depression—can significantly impact communication and connection within our relationships.

• **How Pain Changes Interactions:** If think about it: when we're in pain, we might be less patient, more irritable, or simply less able to participate in activities we used to enjoy together. This can lead to misunderstandings, frustration, and even resentment on both sides. It's easy for those closest to us to feel helpless or unsure how to support or interact with someone in pain, and conversely, it is also quite common for the person experiencing pain to feel isolated, misunderstood, or feel as though they are a burden.

• **Shifting Roles and Responsibilities:** Sometimes, pain can shift roles and responsibilities within our relationships. If pain limits someone's ability to perform certain tasks, their family members or caregivers may need to take on additional responsibilities. This can create imbalances and strain, especially if communication isn't clear and open. It can also be tough for the person in pain to accept help, as it might feel like a loss of independence.

• **Impact on Intimacy and Connection:** It's also important to acknowledge that pain can affect intimacy and our emotional connections in all kinds of relationships. When someone is in pain, interest in social interactions wanes and enjoyable conversations become far less frequent. This can lead to feelings of separation, loneliness, and as sense of disconnection for everyone involved.

• **The Importance of Open Communication:**
We want to also mention that open and honest communication is an important aspect of all our relationships. Whether it's the person experiencing pain or the caregiver and support person, talking about the pain, expressing needs, and acknowledging the emotional impact on everyone involved, helps to build and reinforce a strong foundation for managing all the various aspects of pain and its effect on relationships.

The Emotional Components of Pain:

Next, let's talk about something that's often harder to deal with than the physical pain itself: the emotional roller-coaster that is part of the ride. Consider this; pain isn't just a sensation in our bodies; it's deeply intertwined with our emotions, affecting everything from our mood, our sense of self, and even our thoughts, affecting how we navigate every aspect of our lives. Understanding this pain/emotions/life equation is key to navigating the challenges and reclaiming a sense of well-being. Next, we will take a closer look at the complex, and potent ways pain affects our emotions which can help us understand the far-reaching impacts of pain on our lives.

• **Pain's Emotional Impact:** Pain is not just a physical sensation; it has a profound impact on our emotional well-being. When we experience pain, a range of emotions can arise, including anxiety, frustration, sadness, and anger. These emotions are a natural response to the discomfort and limitations that pain can impose. As discussed in Chapter 7, mindfulness provides a powerful set of tools for working with difficult emotions such as anxiety, frustration, and sadness. These same skills can be applied to the emotional challenges that arise in the context of pain.

• **Pain, Fear, Worry, Anxiety:** Pain can often trigger a cascade of related emotions. Initially, there might be a sense of fear—fear of what the pain means, fear of it getting worse, or fear of the unknown. This fear can then lead to worry—obsessing over the cause of the pain, its potential duration, and its impact on our ability to carry out daily activities. This worry, if left unchecked, can escalate into anxiety, a more pervasive feeling of unease and apprehension. As we previously explored, practicing mindful breathing or body scans can help us ground ourselves in the present moment and reduce the intensity of these anxious feelings, interrupting the cycle of fear, worry, and anxiety.

• **Pain, Frustration, Sadness, and Anger:** When pain persists or interferes with our lives, it's natural to experience a range of challenging emotions. Initially, there might be frustration—a sense of impatience and irritation at not being able to do the things we enjoy or need to do. This frustration, if prolonged or intense, can lead to sadness or even grief as we mourn the loss of physical abilities, independence, or a sense of normalcy. If these feelings of sadness are not acknowledged or processed, they can sometimes morph into anger, directed at the pain itself, at our bodies for "betraying" us, or even at others who may not fully understand our experience.

• **The Challenge of Cyclical Pain:** The emotional impact of pain can be particularly challenging when the pain is cyclical, with periods of increasing intensity, easing, and flare-ups. This unpredictability can create a sense of constant vigilance and anticipatory anxiety, making it difficult to relax and enjoy life. But it's not just the unpredictability of flare-ups that's challenging; it's also the predictability of how certain activities might trigger or worsen the pain. This knowledge forces us to constantly manage our activities, weighing the potential benefits against the risk of increased pain or a prolonged recovery period. For example, someone with chronic back pain might know that gardening for more than an hour will likely lead to increased pain the next day or even a multi-day setback. This constant need for anticipatory management can significantly impact how we live our lives, limiting our spontaneity, requiring careful planning, and sometimes forcing us to give up activities we once enjoyed. The emotional roller coaster of cyclical pain, combined with this constant need for management, can be exhausting and demoralizing.

• **Pain and the Sense of Loss:** Pain can lead to a profound sense of loss, impacting not only our physical abilities but also our sense of who we are. It's not just about losing the ability to do certain activities; it's about the loss of the self that was able to do those things. This can be one of the most difficult aspects of living with chronic pain.

• **Loss of previous activities:** If you were once an avid gardener and now find it difficult to even bend over, you might feel a loss not just of your gardening hobby but also of your identity as a gardener. If you were once a marathon runner and now struggle to walk around the block, you might feel a loss of your identity as an athlete. These losses can be deeply felt, triggering a grieving process similar to mourning the loss of a loved one.

Loss of Sense of Self

This loss of self can manifest in various ways. It might be a loss of independence, as we become reliant on others for help with daily tasks. It might be a loss of social connection, as pain limits our ability to participate in social activities. It might be a loss of purpose, as pain disrupts our work, hobbies, or other meaningful pursuits. And perhaps most significantly, it can be a loss of a sense of control over our own bodies and lives.

This sense of loss can be incredibly painful and isolating. It's important to acknowledge these feelings and allow ourselves to grieve the changes that pain has brought to our lives. *It's also essential to remember that you are not alone, and seeking support is a sign of strength.* This support can come from various sources, including family, friends, support groups, faith communities, healthcare providers, and mental health professionals.

It's important to note:

If you are experiencing thoughts of hopelessness, despair, or even thoughts of harming yourself, please know that help is available. Please reach out to a trusted friend, family member, healthcare provider, or mental health professional immediately. You can also call the 988 Suicide & Crisis Lifeline in the United States by dialing 988 or visiting **988lifeline.org**.

These feelings of loss are explored in Chapter 9, which discusses grief and loss in the context of aging. For a more in-depth exploration of mindfulness techniques for managing difficult emotions, please refer to Chapter 7.

IV. Our Unique Relationship to Pain

Individual Differences in Pain Perception

Consider this...No two people are exactly alike. We each have our own unique genetic makeup, life experiences, emotional landscape, and ways of coping with challenges. It only makes sense, then, that our experience of pain would also be unique. What feels like a minor twinge to one person might be truly debilitating for another, and vice-versa.

This isn't a matter of weakness or strength; it's simply a reflection of our individual differences. There's no "right" or "wrong" way to experience pain. Your experience is your experience, and it's OK no matter what your experience of, or relationship to pain is. These individual perceptions are shaped by a complex interplay of factors, which we'll explore in more detail below.

Pain Threshold vs. Pain Tolerance:

To really understand why pain is so different for everyone, it helps to look at two key concepts: pain threshold and pain tolerance.

Think of your pain threshold as the point where you first start to notice a sensation as being painful—like the first flicker of heat when you touch something warm. This threshold tends to be fairly similar from person to person.

While, pain tolerance—how much of that sensation you can endure—is a different story. This is where things get really personal. Here are some things that can influence our pain tolerance:

- **The Mind's Influence:** Our mental and emotional state significantly influences our experience of pain. Psychological factors such as anxiety, fear, and catastrophizing (when we tend to imagine the worst possible outcome) can actually amplify the pain signals our bodies send. For instance, if you're already feeling anxious about a doctor's appointment, even a routine examination might feel more uncomfortable than usual.

- **Thoughts, Beliefs, and Pain:** Our thoughts and beliefs about pain directly influence our experience. If we constantly tell ourselves things like "I can't handle this" or "This will never get better," it can create a cycle of negativity that makes the pain feel even worse. On the other hand, cultivating more helpful thoughts and developing effective coping strategies can make a real difference in how we manage pain.

Other Influencing Factors: Several other factors also contribute to these individual differences:

- **Personality and Coping Styles:** Some of us are naturally more resilient and have developed more effective ways of coping with challenging situations, including pain. For instance, someone with a strong sense of self-efficacy (belief in their ability to handle challenges) might be better equipped to manage pain than someone who tends to feel helpless in the face of adversity.

• **Cultural and Social Influences:** Our cultural background and social environment can shape our beliefs and expectations about pain, influencing how we express and manage it.

• **Past Experiences:** What we've experienced in the past with pain can certainly color how we perceive current pain.

• **Physical Health and Existing Conditions:** Our overall physical health and any existing health conditions can also play a role in how we experience pain and how our bodies heal.

It's important to remember that these factors often interact with each other, creating a unique and complex pain experience for each individual.

V. Integrating Mindfulness with Other Pain Management Approaches

Mindfulness can be a valuable tool in managing pain, particularly when dealing with moderate to severe pain. It's important to remember that mindfulness is most effective when integrated with other appropriate pain management strategies and under the guidance of your healthcare provider. While mindfulness can be helpful for mild pain as well, it's often in cases of more persistent or intense pain that a multi-faceted approach, combining mindfulness with other treatments, becomes most beneficial.

Working with Healthcare Providers: The most important aspect of integrating mindfulness is open communication with your healthcare team. Discuss your interest in using mindfulness with your doctor, physical therapist, or other healthcare professionals. They can help you determine if mindfulness is appropriate for your specific condition and can help you integrate it with other treatments you may be receiving.

Other Pain Management Techniques: There are many other effective pain management approaches, including physical therapy, medication, injections, and other medical interventions. Mindfulness can complement these approaches by helping you manage the emotional and mental aspects of pain, reduce stress, and improve your overall well-being. This chapter does not go into detail about these other approaches, as they are best discussed with your healthcare provider. Other complementary approaches, such as acupuncture, massage therapy, and other mind-body techniques, may also be helpful for some individuals. It's important to discuss any complementary treatments with your healthcare provider to ensure they are appropriate for your specific situation and don't interact negatively with other treatments you are receiving.

Medication Dependence and Mindfulness: In some cases, mindfulness can help reduce reliance on medication for pain management, but this should always be done in consultation with your doctor. Never change or stop taking prescribed medication without first discussing it with your healthcare provider. Mindfulness can be a helpful tool in managing pain and improving quality of life, but it is not a replacement for medical care.

VI. Our Complex Relationships with Pain

Acceptance and Resistance

How do you see pain? As a burden or annoyance? Perhaps an opponent? Maybe even a teacher? Our relationships with pain are as varied and unique as we are. Sometimes, we meet pain with acceptance, learning from it and finding ways to integrate it into our lives. But often, and perhaps more commonly, we resist it. We push it away, fight against it, and try to ignore it.

This resistance, while understandable, can actually make our experience of pain more difficult. In this section, we're going to explore the many ways we resist pain—some obvious, others more subtle—and how understanding these patterns can open the door to a more functional, tolerant, calmer, and accepting relationship with your own unique experience of pain.

Mental Resistance:

You can probably relate to this... It's the big emphatic "No, no, no!" that our brain throws up into our awareness when it comes to pain. It's human nature to want to avoid pain—both physical and mental. So, it's no surprise that one of the most common ways we resist pain is in our minds. This mental resistance can take many forms, from simply trying to distract ourselves to actively suppressing any thoughts or feelings related to the pain. It might show up as:

• **Distraction:** Constantly engaging in activities to keep the mind occupied and avoid thinking about pain.

• **Suppression:** Consciously pushing away any thoughts or feelings related to pain.

• **Denial:** Refusing to acknowledge the experience or severity of pain.

• **Rumination (in reverse):** Obsessively focusing on the negative aspects of pain, catastrophizing about the future, and replaying past painful experiences.

This mental avoidance, can actually exacerbate pain in the long run. By not acknowledging and processing our pain, we prevent ourselves from developing effective coping strategies which can create a cycle of anxiety and fear that amplifies the our experience of the pain.

Cultural Resistance:

We all grow up surrounded by messages about pain, often from our families, communities, and the wider culture. These messages can shape how we think about pain and how we react to it. For example, we might hear things like "Be strong," "Don't be a baby," or "Just tough it out." These kinds of messages can create a cultural pressure to suppress or minimize pain, making us feel like showing vulnerability is a sign of weakness. This cultural resistance can manifest in several ways:

- **Stoicism:** Adopting a "grin and bear it" attitude, refusing to acknowledge or express pain, even when it's significant. This is often seen in cultures that value emotional restraint and self-reliance.

- **Minimization:** Downplaying the severity of pain, perhaps saying things like "It's just a little ache" or "I'm fine," even when experiencing considerable discomfort.

- **Exaggeration (for attention):** On the opposite end of the spectrum, some cultural contexts might inadvertently encourage exaggerating pain to gain attention or sympathy. This can become a learned behavior, even if the initial pain was minor.

These cultural influences can create a complex internal conflict. We might feel pressure to conform to societal expectations, even if it means ignoring our own needs and making our pain worse. Mindfulness can help us become aware of these cultural messages and choose a more authentic response to pain, one that honors both our individual experience and our need for support.

Emotional Resistance:

Let's be real, pain isn't just about what's happening in our bodies; it hits us in our hearts and minds too. When pain sticks around or gets really intense, it can stir up a whole bunch of tough emotions—fear, anxiety, frustration, anger, sadness, you name it. It's like a chain reaction: the pain triggers the emotions, and those emotions can make the pain feel even worse.

It's totally understandable that we might want to resist these feelings, to push them away or numb them out. This emotional resistance can show up in lots of different ways:

- **Emotional numbing:** Shutting down our emotions to avoid feeling the full impact of the pain. This can lead to a sense of detachment from ourselves and others.

- **Avoidance of situations that might trigger pain:** This might involve avoiding activities we once enjoyed, social interactions, or even medical appointments, leading to isolation and a diminished quality of life.

- **Hopelessness and despair:** Feeling overwhelmed by the pain and believing that it will never get better. This can lead to a sense of helplessness and a loss of motivation to engage in self-care or seek support.

- **Irritability and anger:** Feeling constantly on edge and reacting with anger or frustration to even minor inconveniences. This can strain relationships and create further emotional distress.

As we explored in Chapter 7: Mindfulness for Emotional and Mental Well-being, our emotions play a significant role in our overall experience, and this is especially true when dealing with pain.

Suppressing or avoiding emotions can actually intensify the experience of pain and make it more difficult to manage.

Mindfulness can help us gently acknowledge and accept these difficult emotions without judgment, allowing us to process them in a healthier way and break free from this cycle of pain > pain resistance > more pain.

Physical Resistance:

And as if mental, cultural, and emotional resistance weren't enough... Sometimes, our resistance to pain is far more basic—something that isn't a matter of choice or conscious effort; it's resistance that is rooted in physical changes in our bodies.

These changes can alter how we perceive pain, sometimes diminishing or even blocking pain signals altogether.

This unique type of resistance can happen for a variety of reasons, many of which are beyond our control:

• **Nerve damage:** Injuries or conditions like neuropathy can damage nerves, disrupting the transmission of pain signals to the brain. This can result in numbness, tingling, or a reduced ability to feel pain in the affected area.

• **Scar tissue:** Scar tissue, which forms after injury or surgery, can sometimes compress nerves or block pain receptors, reducing sensitivity in the area.

• **Brain changes:** In some cases, changes in brain structure or function due to stroke, trauma, or other conditions can affect how pain signals are processed. This can lead to difficulties interpreting pain, or even a complete inability to feel certain types of pain.

• **Congenital Insensitivity to Pain (CIP):** This is a rare genetic condition where a person is born unable to feel physical pain. While it might seem like a blessing, it's actually a very dangerous condition, as pain serves as a vital warning system for our bodies.

It's important to understand that these physical changes are different from the mental, cultural, and emotional forms of resistance we've discussed. In these cases, the resistance isn't about avoiding or suppressing pain; it's about the body's ability to perceive pain being altered.

While mindfulness cannot reverse these physical changes, it can be helpful for managing any associated anxiety or distress. It can also help people with diminished pain sensation to be more attuned to other bodily sensations that might indicate injury or illness.

Other Impactful Influences on Pain Perception:

We often turn to medications to help manage pain, and thankfully, many are very effective at reducing discomfort and improving our quality of life. But it's important to be aware that some impactful influences can alter our awareness of pain and other bodily sensations.

These influences include certain medications (especially strong pain relievers like opioids), alcohol, medicinal or recreational cannabis, other recreational drugs, and even emerging trends like micro-dosing with hallucinogenic substances.

It's not that we're intentionally resisting the pain; it's that our ability to perceive it is being altered by these influences. This altered sensory experience can present some significant health risks and challenges:

- **Masking important signals:** Pain serves as a vital warning system, alerting us to potential injuries or illnesses. If our pain awareness is significantly reduced, we might not notice new injuries or worsening conditions.

• **Increased risk of injury:** If we can't feel pain properly, we might engage in activities that could cause further harm without realizing it. This is especially important to consider with activities that involve heat, cold, or strenuous physical exertion.

• **Potential for overuse or dependence:** In some cases, the desire to avoid any sensation of pain or discomfort can lead to overuse or dependence on these substances, which can have its own set of risks and side effects.

• **Specific considerations for micro-dosing and other emerging trends:** It's important to note that research on the long-term effects of micro-dosing and other less conventional approaches to pain management is still limited. While some individuals report positive experiences, these practices are not yet widely accepted within the medical community and may carry potential risks. It is crucial to consult with a qualified healthcare professional before considering any of these approaches. Self-treating with unregulated substances can be dangerous.

It's crucial to work closely with your healthcare provider or other qualified professional to find the right balance between managing pain or other symptoms and maintaining appropriate body awareness. This is especially true if you are using any medications or substances regularly.

Mindfulness can be a valuable tool in this process:

By cultivating greater body awareness, we can become more attuned to subtle sensations and avoid relying solely on substances to manage pain or discomfort. Mindfulness can also help us develop alternative coping strategies that can reduce our reliance on medication or other substances over time.

When to Seek Professional Help:

While mindfulness can be a powerful tool for working with and managing pain, it's crucial to recognize when professional medical attention is necessary. Seeking help can prevent further injury or tissue damage and address underlying causes of pain that are beyond self-management.

Remember, seeking help is a sign of strength, self-awareness, and a commitment to your well-being. Here are some general guidelines for when it is appropriate to seek additional pain support:

- **Sudden or severe pain:** If you experience sudden, intense pain that is unlike anything you've felt before, seek immediate medical attention. This could be a sign of a serious underlying condition.

- **Pain that interferes with daily life:** If pain is significantly impacting your ability to work, sleep, eat, or engage in other daily activities, it's time to consult a healthcare professional.

• **Persistent or worsening pain:** If pain persists for more than a few weeks or gradually worsens over time, even if it's not initially severe, it's important to seek medical advice.

• **Pain accompanied by other symptoms:** If your pain is accompanied by other concerning symptoms, such as fever, swelling, numbness, tingling, weakness, changes in bowel or bladder function, chest pain, shortness of breath, dizziness, extremity numbness (especially on one side of the body), speech changes, vision changes, throbbing sensations (especially in the head or neck), or sudden profuse sweating, consult a healthcare professional promptly or dial 911 (or your local emergency number).

• **Pain that doesn't respond to self-care measures:** If you've tried self-care measures like rest, gentle stretching, or over-the-counter pain relievers and your pain doesn't improve or gets worse, it's time to seek professional help.

• **Emotional distress related to pain:** If your pain is causing significant emotional distress, such as anxiety, depression, hopelessness, or especially if you are experiencing suicidal thoughts, it's crucial to seek immediate support. Contact a mental health professional, discuss your concerns with your healthcare provider, or call 988 (the Suicide & Crisis Lifeline) or your local emergency number.

Remember, every person's experience with pain is unique. If you have any concerns about your pain, it's always best to err on the side of caution and consult with a healthcare professional. They can provide a proper diagnosis, recommend appropriate treatment options, and help you develop a comprehensive pain management plan.

VII. Examples and Success Stories

While every person's experience with pain is unique, these anonymized examples illustrate how mindfulness techniques can be helpful in managing and working with different types of pain:

• **Chronic Back Pain:** Sarah had been living with chronic back pain for years. It affected her sleep, her ability to work, and her overall mood. Through mindfulness techniques, she learned to observe the sensations of pain without judgment, noticing the changing intensity and location of the discomfort. This awareness helped her to create space between the pain and her reactions to it, reducing her anxiety and allowing her to engage more fully in daily activities.

• **Post-Surgical Pain:** John experienced significant pain after knee surgery. He used mindfulness techniques, such as body scans and mindful breathing, to focus on the present moment and manage the intensity of the pain. By focusing on his breath and observing the sensations in his body, he was able to reduce his reliance on pain medication and improve his recovery process.

• **Migraine Headaches:** Maria suffered from frequent and debilitating migraine headaches. She began practicing mindfulness meditation, focusing on the sensations in her body and the thoughts that arose during a headache. Through regular engagement with mindfulness techniques, she noticed that she was able to recognize the early warning signs of a migraine and implement strategies, such as rest and mindful breathing, to reduce the severity and duration of her headaches.

• **Post-Traumatic Pain (Non-Surgical):** After a car accident, David experienced persistent neck and shoulder pain, even though he hadn't required surgery. The pain was accompanied by anxiety and difficulty sleeping. He began practicing mindfulness techniques, including mindful movement and guided imagery, to help him reconnect with his body and manage the physical and emotional effects of the trauma. By focusing on gentle movements and visualizing peaceful scenes, he was able to reduce his pain levels, improve his sleep, and lessen his anxiety.

These examples are randomized and fictionalized they do reflect common strategies experiences that people have used. They illustrate that mindfulness is not a magic cure, but a tool that can help individuals develop a different relationship with pain, reducing its impact on their lives.

VIII. Chapter 8 Exercises

Mindfulness Techniques and Approaches for Pain Management:

Now that we've explored the various types of physical pain, as well as the mental and emotional aspects of pain, let's dive into some practical mindfulness techniques that can help us work directly with these challenging sensations. Remember, the goal isn't to eliminate the pain but to change our relationship with it, allowing us to experience it with greater awareness and acceptance.

This section offers a variety of mindfulness techniques. You can explore each one and choose the approaches that feel most helpful and accessible to you. There is no one-size-fits-all approach to mindfulness, and it's important to find what works best for your individual needs and preferences.

A Note on Pain Levels:

While mindfulness can be helpful for many people experiencing pain, it's important to acknowledge that working with severe pain can be particularly challenging. If you are experiencing severe pain, it's essential to consult with your healthcare provider to develop an appropriate pain management plan. Mindfulness can then be used as a complementary approach alongside other medical treatments.

Foundational Mindfulness for Pain: Noticing and Relaxing

There are 5 exercises that follow:

• The first 3 (exercises 1, 2, and 3 below) are techniques that can be helpful for managing and working with your discomfort and pain.

• The last 2 (exercises 4 and 5 below), present two techniques to directly meet your pain, without trying to change the experience of the pain perception.

Here are some ways you can use the exercises that follow:

• **You mix and match** the following exercises as you are so inclined

• **You can engage in one or more** of the first 3 before moving on to the last two (this approach can calm your pain and ease any tension)

• **You can do any of the first three during or after** the last two exercises to help regulate your emotions and promote relaxation.

Each of these techniques are valuable tools in their own right and can be used anytime, even when you're not experiencing acute pain. Please use these exercises in any way that you feel drawn.

Mindful Breathing & Pain:

Mindful breathing is a cornerstone of many formal and informal mindfulness approaches, and can be especially helpful when dealing with pain. When we experience pain, our breathing can become shallow and rapid, which can exacerbate feelings of anxiety and tension. Mindful breathing helps us regulate our breath, promoting relaxation and a sense of calm, which can, in turn, reduce the perceived intensity of pain. This simple act can anchor us in the present moment, reduce our "pain story" narrative, and reduce negative self-talk or catastrophizing by providing a sense of calm, an inner stability, and a less reactive state during times of discomfort.

Exercise 1 for Meeting and Managing Pain —Mindful Breathing

- **Find a comfortable position,** either sitting or lying down. You can close your eyes or keep them softly open.

- **Bring your awareness to your breath.** Notice the sensation of the air entering and leaving your body. You might feel the rise and fall of your chest or abdomen, or the gentle flow of air through your nostrils.

- **Simply Observe.** There's no need to change your breath in any way; simply observe it as it is. Is it shallow? Deep? Fast? Or slow?

- **As you breathe,** you might notice your mind wandering. This is perfectly normal. When you notice your attention drifting, gently redirect it back to the sensation of your breath.

• **Continue this gentle observation** of your breath for a few minutes. If your attention is drawn to the pain, gently acknowledge it without judgment and then redirect your focus back to your breath. Notice how your body feels with each breath. Does the pain feel any different as you breathe deeply and calmly?

• **Gently Ending.** When you're ready, slowly open your eyes (if they were closed) and end with a few calm mindful breaths.

• **Take a moment to notice how you feel.** Do you notice any difference in your pain or how you feel about your pain? There's no need for anything to have changed; simply notice what you are sensing.

Mindful Movement & Pain:

When we are in pain, we may become less active, which can lead to stiffness and increased discomfort. Mindful movement involves bringing awareness to the sensations of movement in the body, paying attention to each movement as it unfolds, within a pain-free range of motion. This can help release tension, improve circulation, and gently encourage movement in areas affected by pain.

This can be as simple as gentle stretching or swaying, walking, just moving your fingers and toes, or engaging in yoga or tai chi or other mindful slow exercise. **It's crucial to move within your pain-free range of motion.** This means moving only to the point where you feel a gentle stretch or sensation, but not so much as to increase your pain.

If a movement causes pain, stop immediately and gently return to a resting position. Remember to stay within your pain-free range of motion and a comfortable pain-free activity level.

Exercise 2 for Meeting & Managing Pain —Mindful Movement

- **Begin by finding a comfortable position** (standing or seated).

- **Bring your awareness to your body.** Notice any sensations of tension or stiffness.

- **Begin to move your body gently.** You might start by slowly rotating your head, shrugging your shoulders, or gently stretching your arms and legs.

- **Pay close attention to the sensations in your body.** Notice how each movement feels.

    ◇ Are there any areas of tightness or resistance?

    ◇ You might choose to simply pause and rest at that point, gently observing the sensations in that area without pushing into the pain.

◇ Pay attention to how the pain feels as you move.

◇ Does it lessen, stay the same, or increase? Remember to stay within your pain-free range of motion.

◇ Notice any areas of tension that might be contributing to your pain.

◇ As you move, see if you can gently release some of that tension.

• **Move slowly and deliberately,** coordinating your movements with your breath.

• **If you experience any increase in pain,** stop the movement and gently return to a resting position. You can then try a smaller, gentler movement.

• **Continue this mindful movement for a few minutes,** exploring different movements as you feel comfortable.

• **Gently Ending.** When you are ready, slowly stop your movement, take a few mindful breaths, return you awareness to your surroundings.

• **Take a moment to notice how you feel.** Do you notice any difference in your pain or how you feel about your pain?

There's no need for anything to have changed; simply notice what is present.

Music, Sound & Pain:

Music and sound can have a profound impact on our mood and our experience of pain. Mindful listening involves bringing focused attention to the sounds around us or to music we choose to listen to. This can help shift our focus away from pain, promote relaxation, and create a sense of calm, which can indirectly influence our perception of pain.

Exercise 3: Meeting and Managing Pain —Mindful Sounds

• **Find a comfortable position,** either sitting or lying down.

• **Choose some calming music or...** simply bring your awareness to the sounds around you.

• **Begin to listening to the music or sounds.** Immerse yourself in sound source or soundscape. Notice the different instruments, melodies, rhythms, or the different qualities and duration of the sounds around you.

• **If your mind wanders**, gently bring your attention back to the sounds.

• **As you listen, notice if the music or sounds have any effect on your pain or discomfort,** or any associated tension, worry, anxiety, or stress. Do they help you feel more relaxed or distracted from the pain?

• **Continue this mindful listening** for a few minutes.

(Exercise continues next page)

• **Return to our surroundings.** Take a few mindful breaths as you begin to return to your surroundings.

• **Take a few moment to reflect on how you feel now.** Do you notice any difference in your pain or how you feel about your pain?

There's no need for anything to have changed; simply notice what is present.

Mindfulness & Working with Pain

The following two exercises aren't about trying to modulate your pain and change it in anyway; it's about getting to know it better.

Often, our instinct is to push pain away, to resist it. But by gently turning our attention toward the sensations, we can learn valuable information about its nature.

This can help us develop a different relationship with our aches and pains, including a gentle self-inquiry curiosity, non-critical acceptance, and calmer responses, as opposed to strong reactions, resistance and anxiety.

Exercise 4 for Meeting and Managing Pain —Mindful Explorations of Pain

• **Find a comfortable position,** either sitting or lying down. Gently close your eyes or soften your gaze.

- **Bring your awareness to your body.** Simply notice any sensations without bias or judgment.

- **Gently direct your attention** to the area of your body where you are experiencing pain.

- **Notice the qualities of the pain.** Instead of focusing on the intensity of the pain, try to notice other aspects such as; Where exactly is it located? Is it a sharp, dull, burning, or aching sensation? Does it feel constant or intermittent? Is the pain moving? Are there any other sensations such as tightness, heat, tingling, or throbbing?

- **Simply observe your sensations** with gentle curiosity, as if you were exploring a new landscape. There's no need to change anything; just notice what's there.

- **If your mind wanders,** gently redirect your attention back to the sensations in your body.

- **Continue this gentle observation** for a few minutes.

- **Return to your surroundings.** When you're ready, gently take a few mindful breathes and slowly open your eyes.

- **Take a moment to notice how you feel.** Do you notice any difference in your pain or how you feel about your pain?

Once again, there's no need for anything to have changed; simply notice what is present.

Sensory Awareness of Pain

This technique builds upon the "Find the Pain" Exercise, taking our exploration of pain sensations a bit deeper. Instead of just locating the pain, we'll focus on the specific sensory qualities associated with it.

This helps us to become more familiar with the ever-changing nature of pain and can help reduce our tendency to be critical or resist it. By focusing on these specific sensory details, we can begin to deconstruct the often overwhelming experience of pain into smaller, more manageable components.

Exercise 5 for Meeting and Managing Pain —Mindful Pain Awareness

- **Find a comfortable position,** either sitting or lying down. Gently close your eyes or soften your gaze.

- **Bring your awareness to the area of your body** where you are experiencing pain.

- **Begin to pay close attention** to the specific sensations you are experiencing. Try to describe them to yourself using descriptive words. For example:

  ◇ **Location:** Where exactly is the pain located? Is it localized to one spot or does it spread to other areas?

  ◇ **Temperature:** Does it feel hot, cold, warm, or neutral?

◇ **Texture:** Does it feel sharp, dull, throbbing, aching, burning, tingling, tight, or numb?

◇ **Movement:** Does the pain feel constant, intermittent, or pulsating? Does it move or shift?

◇ **Fluctuations:** While we're not focusing on rating the overall intensity of the pain, you might notice that the sensation changes or fluctuates. Simply observe these changes without judgment.

• **As you observe these sensations,** try to maintain an attitude of curiosity and acceptance. There's no need to change anything; simply notice what's there, moment by moment.

• **If your mind wanders,** gently redirect your attention back to the sensations in your body.

• **Continue this focused observation** for a few minutes.

• **Return to your surroundings.** When you're ready, with a few gently mindful breaths, slowly open your eyes.

• **Take a moment to notice how you feel.** Do you notice any difference in your pain or how you feel about your pain?

There's no need for anything to have changed; simply notice what is present.

IX. Chapter 8 Conclusion

This chapter has explored the complex and multifaceted nature of pain, moving beyond the simplistic view of it as a purely physical experience. We've seen how pain is deeply intertwined with our thoughts, emotions, cultural influences, and personal experiences. A key theme has been the concept of resistance—how our natural tendency to push away or fight against pain can often intensify our suffering, creating a vicious cycle.

Mindfulness offers a powerful alternative to this cycle of resistance. By cultivating present moment awareness and a relaxed, gentle, and kind-to-ourselves observation, we can learn to relate to pain in a new way. Mindfulness helps us create space between the sensation and our reactions, allowing us to respond with greater wisdom and compassion rather than reactivity and fear.

It's crucial to remember that mindfulness is one component of a holistic approach to pain management. Recognizing when professional medical or mental health support is necessary is a sign of strength and self-awareness. Combining mindfulness with appropriate medical care, and exploring complementary approaches (as we discuss in the upcoming *Chapter 10: Bringing Mindfulness into Your Life*), can empower you to manage pain more effectively.

X. Looking Ahead to Chapter 9: Mindfulness for Grief, Loss, and Life Transitions

In Chapter 9 we will turn our attention to the last of our Life Challenges chapters presenting another area where mindful exercises and techniques can be extremely helpful: the areas of Grief, Loss, and Life Transitions. The following chapter examines in depth the various aspects of these difficult experiences and how these the same mindfulness approaches and principles can be applied to manage both the emotional and physical responses that associated with grief, loss, and life transitions.

Chapter 9

"Grief is the price we pay for love."

Queen Elizabeth II

"You have to keep breaking your heart
until it opens."

Rumi

"The art of living lies less in eliminating
our troubles than in growing with them."

Bernard M. Baruch

CHAPTER LEVEL TABLE OF CONTENTS

Chapter 9: Mindfulness for Grief, Loss, and Life Transitions

Chapter 9

Mindfulness for Grief, Loss, and Life Transitions

Another Long Chapter Ahead:

There is a lot of information to present when discussing grief, loss, life transitions and our relationships to them. Again, I have endeavored to keep the explanations as simple as possible while also trying to relay both relevant and helpful information. Take your time with this chapter as it touches on several very important and challenging topics.

I. Introduction

Loss, grief, and life's transitions are among the most challenging life events we face—often profoundly impacting our lives. And navigating these life changes can trigger a wide spectrum of powerful emotions, including sadness, anger, confusion, fear, anxiety, guilt, and more.

The unexpected magnitude of these feelings can present very real challenges to how we experience life and interact with the world. Just as everyone's experience with pain is unique, so too is their relationship to grief and loss.

While mindfulness won't "fix" our emotions or remove our emotional pain, it offers simple, accessible, and effective strategies to navigate these difficult emotions surrounding change and loss. And while riding the waves of extreme emotions may not be "easy," the potential benefits are important to consider.

By engaging with even the simplest mindfulness approaches, such as simple breath awareness or even rudimentary mindful movements—both core mindfulness techniques—we can, in time, learn to lean directly into the experience of difficult emotions with greater ease, calm, and significantly less upheaval or volatility.

This chapter explores, in some depth, the various aspects of grief, loss, and change (life transitions) and presents several mindful approaches that can support you through these kinds of emotional challenges, helping you regain emotional stability, even when emotions are running fast and furious.

II. Defining & Understanding Loss, Grief, and Life Transitions:

To understand how mindfulness can support us through these difficult times, it's crucial to explore the complexities of loss, grief, and the transitions they bring. First, some definitions:

236

Loss refers to the experience of no longer having something or someone valued.

• Loss takes many forms. While the death of a loved one is often the first thing that comes to mind when we think of grief, loss can encompass a much wider range of experiences. It can be the end of a relationship, the loss of a job or career, a health challenge that alters our abilities or sense of well-being, the loss of a treasured possession, or even the transition from one life stage to another— from childhood to adolescence, from singlehood to parenthood, or from working life to retirement. Each of these experiences, while vastly different in their specifics, shares a common thread: the loss of something valued, something familiar, something that was a part of our lives.

Grief is the natural emotional response to loss.

• Grief, the emotional response to loss, is equally varied. While the "stages of grief" (denial, anger, bargaining, depression, and acceptance) are frequently discussed, it's crucial to understand that grief is not a linear progression through these stages. People may experience these emotions in different orders, revisit certain emotions multiple times, or not experience some of them at all. Grief is a deeply personal and often unpredictable journey.

Life transitions are periods of significant change.

• Life transitions, even those that are generally considered positive, can also trigger emotional responses similar to those experienced during grief. Moving to a new city, starting a new job, or becoming a parent can bring about feelings of loss for the familiar routines, relationships, and sense of identity associated with our previous circumstances. These transitions, while often exciting, can also be challenging as we adjust to new realities and let go of the past.

• Importantly, life transitions also encompass the ultimate transition: death itself. Confronting our own mortality can be a profound and often challenging experience, bringing with it a dizzying range of complex and profound emotions.

Six Common Responses to Grief, Loss, and Life Transitions

Throughout all of these experiences—grief, loss, and life transitions—there are generally considered to be six options for how this will play out: personal overwhelm, fear, drama, anger, numbing, and resignation *(While further research is needed to formally categorize these responses, they are based on my own observations, perceptions and experiences working with individuals facing grief and loss as well as with conversations with mental health professionals).*

III. The Role of Mindfulness in Navigating Grief, Loss, and Life Transitions

Grief, loss, or significant life changes are some of our most profoundly difficult and potentially life-altering emotions. Tactics such as minimizing, gritting our teeth and enduring them, or even attempting to entirely block out these strong emotions with denial or substances is not that uncommon.

Enter the supportive framework of mindfulness. A gentle approach to help navigate turbulent emotions, whether one uses a traditional "practice" approach or a simpler as-needed and on-demand strategy. Mindfulness gives us the tools to safely experience our emotions without being derailed or overwhelmed.

The Two Key Elements of a Mindful Approach

Mindfulness and Non-Biased Acceptance: A key aspect of mindfulness is its emphasis on acknowledging and gently accepting difficult emotions without bias or agenda (often referred to as non-judgment or non-judgmental acceptance).

When faced with painful feelings, as previously mentioned, our natural tendency is to seek ease or respite from the emotions, push them away, drown them out, or distract ourselves in one way or another. However, resistance to emotions can have the opposite effect, intensifying our reactions and our suffering.

The mindfulness approach we present encourages us to gently turn toward our emotions in the spirit of self-curiosity and relaxed openness, mindfully observing their arising and subsiding without getting caught up in their drama or swept away by emotional upheaval.

This acceptance doesn't mean we have to like or enjoy our challenging emotions; it means we simply acknowledge their presence without actively adding layers of judgment, blame, or self-criticism (negative self-talk).

Mindfulness and Present Moment Awareness:
Without a doubt, the most important aspects of mindfulness lie in its techniques and strategies that allow us to settle into our present-moment experience.

Despite the simplicity, it is this present-moment awareness that can be the "life raft" that buoys in our moments of upset. A life raft that allows us to ride the undulating waves of thought and emotion, and keep us from drowning in a sea of our own ruminations about the past and future.

If left unchecked, our autopilot reactions (thinking and emotional patterns) have the capacity to lock us into endless cycles of mental and emotional distress.

The good news is that even the simplest and most basic of techniques, such as focusing on a single breath, simple and gentle body movements, or a momentary focus on body sensations, can reset our and ground our upset, allowing us to settle into the here and now.

A Flexible Strategy

Throughout the various emotions that arise during times of loss and change, mindfulness offers a flexible, adaptable, and supportive approach for calming self-care and self-compassion that is both life-affirming, and supportive of personal growth and transformation.

Even in the face of enormous emotional challenges, mindfulness can act as a supplemental support strategy to complement other medical or mental health treatments.

Mindfulness is a tool that encourages us to listen to our needs, honor our limits, and offer ourselves the same compassion we would offer a dear friend.

In-Depth Content Ahead:

Next, together we'll explore the different faces of grief, loss, and life transitions and how they can impact our lives and sense of well-being. While we have endeavored to keep the explanations as simple as possible, there is a lot of information to absorb. Take your time and feel free to read only what you are drawn to, or jump to the exercises at the end of the chapter if you prefer.

IV. Strength, Calm, and Emotional Resilience Through Mindfulness in Times of Loss and Transition

Life inevitably presents us with profoundly difficult experiences—times of significant loss, profound change, and seemingly overwhelming challenges that can test our emotional and mental well-being and rock our foundational sense of self and life-purpose.

This chapter offers guidance on how mindfulness can provide support, foster emotional strength, and offer a path to comfort, ease, and healing during these difficult experiences. We will explore specific contexts, such as grief after the loss of a loved one, relationship endings, job transitions, and health challenges, offering tailored mindfulness techniques and exercises (see end of this chapter) to help you navigate these experiences with greater awareness, insight, self-compassion, and inner strength.

Grief and Loss of Loved Ones:

Loss of a Spouse or Life Partner:

The loss of a spouse or life partner, whether through separation, divorce, or their passing, is a profoundly life-altering event. It's the loss of a constant companion, a confidant, a shared history, and often a significant part of one's daily routine, identity, and future dreams. The grief that follows can be intense and complex, encompassing a wide range of emotions, including profound sadness, loneliness, anger, confusion, disbelief, guilt, and even a sense of being lost or disoriented.

Grief after the loss of a spouse or life partner is a deeply personal journey, and there is no prescribed path. The intensity and duration of grief can vary greatly, and it's important to be patient with yourself and your emotions during this difficult time.

Emotional Considerations: No matter the reason or situation around this difficult situation, the emotional and practical challenges of losing a spouse are often intertwined. The deep sadness, emptiness, and longing that are so common can make even simple daily tasks feel overwhelming. These intense emotions, often experienced in waves of grief, can be physically and emotionally draining, impacting sleep, appetite, and concentration.

As you begin to navigate life without your partner, you may also experience anxiety, fear about the future, a sense of lost purpose, and a feeling of general life disorientation. Whether you are overwhelmed with emotions, surprised by the influx of memories long-forgotten, or choose to intentionally contemplate your past shared experiences, it is all a part of the complex process of healing, adjustment, and moving on with life in a new way.

Practical Considerations: Beyond the emotional impact, there are often many significant practical challenges that arise and need to be navigated. These can include:

• **Changes in daily routines:** Simple everyday tasks that were once shared, such as preparing meals, managing household chores, or making decisions, may now feel overwhelming.

• **Financial adjustments:** Managing finances alone can be stressful, especially if your partner handled those responsibilities. This can add to the emotional burden of grief.

• **Legal and administrative matters:** Dealing with legal paperwork, estate settlements, insurance claims, and other administrative tasks can add to the burden of grief and require significant time and energy.

• **Social adjustments:** Changes in social dynamics and a sense of loneliness can be challenging as you adjust to life without your partner. You may find that social events and gatherings feel different or that you have less in common with friends who are still in relationships.

It's important to remember that the challenges associated with the feelings and emotions, as well as the practical issues that need to be managed are all part of the process, and whatever your inner landscape gives rise to, is normal, completely valid and something to be honored. Be patient with yourself and allow yourself the time and space you need to grieve this kind of loss. There is no set timeline for grief, and it's okay to seek support from friends, family, support groups, or a grief counselor.

(Supporting Exercises for this chapter start on page 268)

Loss of a Child:

The loss of a child, regardless of the child's age, is an unfathomable loss—a parent's worst nightmare. It shatters the natural order of life and leaves a void that can feel impossible to fill. The grief experienced after the death of a child is often described as the most intense and enduring form of grief, marked by profound sadness, anguish, and a deep sense of injustice. There is no single path through this grief. Your experience is uniquely your own, and it is valid, and important part of your healing, however it unfolds.

Emotional and Social Considerations: The emotional impact of losing a child can be devastating and multifaceted. Parents may experience a wide range of intense emotions, including:

- **Overwhelming grief and despair:** A deep and pervasive sadness that can feel all-consuming.

- **Guilt and self-blame:** Parents may question their actions or decisions, wondering if they could have done something differently.

• **Anger and resentment:** Anger may be directed at the situation, at medical professionals, or even at the child for leaving.

• **Disbelief and denial:** It can be difficult to accept the reality of the loss, leading to feelings of disbelief or denial.

• **Anxiety and fear:** Parents may experience anxiety about the future and fear that something bad will happen to other family members.

• **Impact on family dynamics:** The loss of a child can significantly impact family dynamics, affecting relationships between spouses, siblings, and other family members.

• **Social isolation:** Parents may feel isolated and misunderstood by others who haven't experienced a similar loss.

The grief associated with the loss of a child, no matter the age of the parent or grandparent, can be particularly complex due to the unique bond between parent, grandparent, and child. It's the loss of hopes, dreams, and the promise of a future that will never be.

It's crucial to acknowledge the profound impact this loss has on individuals and families. Seeking support from specialized grief counselors, support groups for bereavement, or other resources designed specifically for this type of loss can be immensely helpful.

Loss of Close Personal Relationships:

The loss of a close personal relationship—whether with a parent, sibling, friend, or cherished pet or animal companion—can be a deeply significant and painful experience. These relationships form the fabric of our lives, providing emotional support, enjoyable companionship, and a sense of belonging within our families and communities. While the dynamics of these relationships differ from those with a spouse or child, the grief experienced can be just as profound and impactful.

Emotional and Relational Considerations: The emotional impact of losing a close personal relationship can be multifaceted and deeply felt. You may experience a range of emotions, including:

* **Sadness and longing:** A deep sense of missing the person or animal and the unique bond you shared. This can include missing their presence, their advice, their laughter, or simply their companionship.

* **Loneliness and isolation:** A feeling of being alone without their support and companionship. This can be particularly pronounced if the relationship was a significant source of social connection.

* **Anger and frustration:** Anger at the situation, at an illness, at the circumstances of the loss, or even at the person or animal for leaving.

- **Guilt and regret:** Questioning if you could have done something differently, said something more, or spent more time together. This is a common part of grief, but it's important to remember that you did the best you could with the information and resources you had at the time.

- **Changes in social dynamics:** The loss of a friend or sibling can alter social circles and family dynamics. You may find that gatherings feel different or that you have less in common with those who shared the relationship.

- **Impact on daily routines:** Daily routines may be disrupted, especially if the person or pet played a significant role in your day-to-day life. This might include missing shared activities, rituals, or simply the presence of the person or animal in your home.

- **Feelings of abandonment** (especially in friendships and estrangements): If the relationship ended abruptly or without closure, you might experience feelings of abandonment, rejection, or unworthiness.

The specific nature of the relationship can also influence the grieving process. For example:

- **The loss of a parent** can bring about feelings of becoming an orphan, regardless of your age.

- **The loss of a sibling** can disrupt family dynamics and evoke feelings of lost shared history.

- **The loss of a close friend** can feel like losing a part of yourself, especially if the friendship was long-lasting and close.

- **The loss of a pet**, while often underestimated by those who haven't experienced it, can be a source of profound grief, as pets are often considered members of the family.

It's always important to honor these feelings and recognize that grief is a natural response to loss. There is no right or wrong way to grieve, and it's important to allow yourself the time and space you need to heal and navigate the loss.

(Supporting Exercises for this chapter start on page 268)

Various Other Forms of Personal Loss

Job Loss or Career Transition:

Our careers, jobs, and workplace interactions often comprise a large part of our adult lives. When we experience the loss of a job or career, or a significant change in our workplace, it can lead to a complex array of distressing emotions and significant life adjustments. The main types of changes in this area are:

- Involuntary job loss due to layoff, termination, or company closure.

- Navigating a planned career transition.

- Entering retirement (whether planned, due to health concerns, or other life events).

These shifts in our work life can trigger a wide range of emotions and practical challenges. Whether these changes are anticipated and welcomed or unanticipated and alarming, they can all bring about unexpected adjustments to daily routines, social connections, and sense of purpose. They can also evoke feelings of uncertainty and anxiety as we step into the unknown.

This section addresses the emotional and practical aspects of involuntary job loss, planned career transitions, and the various circumstances surrounding retirement.

Emotional and Practical Considerations: As we've noted, changes in employment can have a significant and widely varied emotional impact, ranging from feelings of uncertainty and anxiety to more profound feelings of loss and grief. The following outlines some of the most common experiences associated with any job loss or career transition.

Involuntary Job Loss:

In the case of involuntary job loss (layoff, termination, company closure), you may experience:

- **Shock and disbelief:** Difficulty processing the news and accepting the change.

- **Anger and resentment:** Feeling angry at your former employer, the circumstances, or even yourself.

- **Fear and anxiety:** Concerns about finances, finding a new job, and the uncertainty of the future.

• **Sadness and grief:** Grieving the loss of your job, your colleagues, and the routine and structure it provided.

• **Loss of self-esteem and confidence:** Feeling a diminished sense of self-worth and questioning your abilities.

Voluntary Career Transitions:

Even in planned career transitions, you may experience:

• **Excitement and anticipation:** Looking forward to new opportunities and challenges.

• **Anxiety about the unknown:** Uncertainty about whether the new path is the right choice.

• **Self-doubt:** Questioning your abilities to succeed in a new field.

• **Stress of the job search/transition:** The process of searching for a new position or adapting to a new role can be demanding.

Retirement (Planned or Unplanned):

Retirement, whether planned or due to unforeseen circumstances, can bring about its own set of emotional and practical considerations:

• **Loss of routine and structure:** Adjusting to a new daily schedule and a lack of work-related activities.

• **Changes in social connections:** Losing daily contact with colleagues and work-related social interactions.

- **Concerns about finances and healthcare:**
Managing finances and healthcare needs in retirement.

- **Searching for new purpose and meaning:**
Finding new ways to engage and contribute in retirement.

- **Mixed emotions (even in planned retirement):**
Even with planning, retirement can bring about mixed emotions, including excitement, relief, sadness, and a sense of loss.

Practical Considerations (Applicable to All Scenarios): Beyond the emotional impact, there are also significant practical considerations that apply to all types of employment changes:

- **Financial concerns:** Managing finances during a period of unemployment or transition.

- **Job searching and networking:** The process of finding a new job or building new professional connections.

- **Updating skills and resumes:** Preparing for a new career or re-entering the workforce.

- **Adjusting to a new routine:** Adapting to a new work schedule or a lack of one.

It's important to acknowledge that any or all of these feelings and challenges are normal and valid. Whether you're facing involuntary job loss, navigating a voluntary career transition, or entering retirement, it's essential to be patient with yourself and your new situation, seek support from friends, family, career counselors, or support groups, and prioritize your physical and mental well-being.

Loss Due to Health Challenges:

Whether a sudden illness or injury, a chronic condition, or the gradual decline of aging, these experiences can be deeply distressing, profoundly impacting all aspects of our lives—our physical and emotional well-being, our independence, our relationships, and our overall quality of life. This section reviews many of the emotional and practical considerations associated with various health experiences and declining health.

Physical and Emotional Considerations: Each person experiences health challenges in their own unique way, but certain emotional and physical responses are common. The following outlines some of these shared experiences:

• **Physical pain and discomfort:** This can range from mild aches to chronic, debilitating pain.

• **Limitations in physical abilities:** Difficulty with mobility, daily tasks, or engaging in activities you once enjoyed.

• **Changes in body image and self-esteem:** Feeling self-conscious about physical changes or limitations.

• **Fear and anxiety:** Concerns about the future, the progression of an illness, or the possibility of further health complications.

• **Sadness and grief:** Grieving the loss of previous health, abilities, or independence.

• **Frustration and anger:** Feeling frustrated with physical limitations or angry at the situation.

• **Feelings of isolation and loneliness:** Difficulty maintaining social connections due to health limitations.

• **Uncertainty and worry:** Concerns about managing symptoms, treatment options, and the overall impact on your life.

The specific nature of the health challenge often influences how we experience those difficulties. For example:

• **Chronic illness:** Can lead to ongoing physical and emotional challenges, requiring long-term management and adaptation.

• **Injury:** Can result in sudden physical limitations and require rehabilitation and recovery.

• **Aging-related decline:** Can bring about gradual changes in physical and cognitive abilities, requiring adjustments to lifestyle and daily routines.

It's important to acknowledge that these feelings and challenges are normal and valid. It's crucial to be patient with yourself, seek appropriate medical care and support, and prioritize your physical and mental well-being.

(Supporting Exercises for this chapter start on page 268)

Life Changes & Transitions

"The Only Constant in Life Is Change." - Heraclitus

Significant Life Changes, Transitions, & Milestones:

While "change" is a constant in life, our relationship to change, whether large or small, anticipated and welcomed, or unexpected and challenging, here we are focusing on the challenging side of change.

It is said that since the earliest days, humans have preferred routine. It makes us feel in control of our lives and gives us something we can feel we can generally rely on. While not all change and life transitions involve loss in the traditional sense, they all have the common theme of a shift in our world and something that can disrupt our routines, challenge our sense of stability and purpose, and force some significant life adjustments.

This section explores the emotional and practical considerations associated with several significant life transitions, including downsizing or relocating, becoming a grandparent or great-grandparent, and other major life changes.

Emotional and Practical Considerations: These transitions, while often positive, can bring about a wide range of emotional experiences, including:

- **Excitement and anticipation:** Looking forward to new beginnings, new family members, or a more enjoyable living situation.

- **Anxiety and uncertainty:** Concerns about adjusting to a new home, new role as a grandparent, or changes in family dynamics.

- **Stress and overwhelm:** Feeling overwhelmed by the tasks involved in moving, setting up a new home, or managing new responsibilities.

- **Mixed emotions:** Experiencing a combination of positive and negative feelings, such as joy at becoming a grandparent mixed with sadness at children moving further away.

- **A sense of loss** (even in positive transitions): Grieving the loss of familiar routines, a larger home, or established social connections.

- **Identity shifts:** Changes in roles and responsibilities can lead to shifts in identity, such as transitioning from a full-time worker to a grandparent.

It's important to remember that the specific circumstances of each transition can significantly influence our experience. For example:

- **Downsizing or Relocating:** Can involve leaving behind a long-time family home, familiar surroundings, and established social connections. It can also bring about the benefits of a more manageable living space, reduced expenses, or proximity to family.

- **Becoming a Grandparent or Great-Grandparent:** This is a major life milestone that brings about new joys and responsibilities. It can also lead to shifts in family dynamics and relationships with adult children.

- **Other Later-Life Changes:** This could include changes in living arrangements (moving in with family, assisted living), changes in health that impact independence, or the loss of a spouse which necessitates changes to living arrangements.

Practical considerations that often accompany these transitions include:

- **Logistical planning and organization:** Managing the details of the transition, such as selling a home, packing, moving, setting up a new home, or making arrangements for childcare (as a grandparent).

• **Financial adjustments:** Changes in income, expenses, or financial responsibilities related to downsizing, relocating, or providing support to grandchildren.

• **Adjusting to new routines and environments:** Adapting to a smaller living space, a new community, or new family dynamics.

• **Building new support systems:** Establishing new connections and finding support in new environments or roles.

While it's important to acknowledge that these any of these transitions, can be unsettling, upsetting, and challenging. It's crucial to be patient with yourself and others during these times of change, seek support when needed, and allow yourself the time to adjust and adapt to your new situation.

(Supporting Exercises for this chapter start on page 268)

Content Warning:

This next section touching on mortality, can be a challenging topic for many. If you are uncomfortable with this topic, please skip ahead to page

Mindfulness and the Acceptance of Mortality:

Our shared reality of death is a fundamental and universally human experience. It is both a profound mystery veiled in layers of the unknown as well as a concrete expression of our natural life cycle. It touches each of us in deeply unique ways. Whether the journey toward this milestone is a long and gradual decline or a sudden and unexpected event, the direct experience of end-of-life transition is a powerful and often transformative catalyst for everyone involved.

Approaching end-of-life transitions often presents a complex emotional landscape, both for the person passing, as well as family, friends an caregivers, ranging from profound states of gratitude, appreciation, love, and awe to unsettling emotions such as fear, anxiety, personal grief, overwhelming sadness, and regret. Whatever the personal experiences and feelings that arise when facing our own mortality, it's important to remember that all emotions are completely valid, worthy of our respect, and deserve to be held with kindness, compassion, and understanding.

In my own experiences with the loss of friends, family, and work with others navigating their own mortality, I have found mindfulness, with its emphasis on abiding present moment awareness coupled to the natural and easy and open acceptance of the current experience, to be a helpful, gentle, and supportive framework for navigating the complex landscape of deep emotion and feelings during a time of mortality and transition.

A gentle reminder...While mindfulness is a useful tool when approaching and navigating mortality, it should be seen as a complementary tool that can be used in conjunction with other professional medical care and support services. Don't think that mindfulness can eliminate or minimize the pain or grief associated with this kind of loss (though it may offer some degree of emotional ease or even some physical relief), and it certainly doesn't try to provide easy answers to life's deepest mysteries. Rather, mindfulness offer strategies and tools that allows us to be fully present with whatever arises, holding our experiences with self-kindness, a compassionate self-understanding, and deep appreciation of whatever arises.

It's important to acknowledge that many find comfort and strength in their personal beliefs, faith traditions, spiritual practices, or philosophical perspectives. These sources of solace, whether rooted in traditional religions, indigenous practices, personal philosophies, or other forms of spiritual or existential understanding, provide a vital refuge during life's final transition. This book honors and respects the diverse ways individuals find meaning and support, and is simply suggesting that mindfulness can complement and reinforce any preferred approach.

Let me offer my own observations of the many experiences with end-of-life transitions I have witnessed over the years. It is simply this: I have witnessed in the presence of those that are passing, whether earlier or later in their transition phase, what appears to be a gentle shift into a relaxed, and naturally-arising receptive awareness, often without any conscious effort, bringing experiences of profound peace and acceptance and an easy release into the unknown for the one that passing. The key point here, from my perspective, is that there is no need to force any particular mindfulness technique or exercise at this important time; rather, it is about allowing this natural process to unfold with care, grace and dignity.

We also want to honor the significance of this period, not only for the individual but also for their loved ones, family, friends, and community. We encourage a compassionate, kind, and loving approach for both the person who is transitioning and those who are close to them during this deeply meaningful and profoundly moving time. We also recognize and pay tribute to the vital role of caregivers and we offer our deep appreciation and support for their invaluable contributions. It is our hope that the tools presented in this book may be of use to anyone navigating this challenging, yet extraordinarily rich, moving, and potentially transformative experience.

(Supporting Exercises for end-of-life transitions start on page 285)

(Supporting Exercises for end-of-life transitions start on page 285)

End of Mortality-Related Content ~

V. Integrating Mindfulness with Other Support Systems

While mindfulness can be a powerful tool for navigating our grief, our experiences of loss, and our challenging life transitions, it is essential to recognize that it is not a replacement for professional support or other community-based resources. Therapy, counseling, support groups, and other forms of professional guidance offer invaluable expertise and support for processing complex emotions and experiences.

If you are struggling with intense grief, persistent sadness, overwhelming anxiety, or other mental health challenges, please do not hesitate to seek help from a qualified mental health professional. These professionals are trained to provide evidence-based support and guidance tailored to your specific needs.

In addition to professional mental health support, there are many other valuable support systems available, including:

- **12-Step Programs:** These programs offer peer support and guidance for individuals struggling with addiction or other behavioral challenges.

- **Peer Support Groups:** These groups provide a safe and supportive space for individuals who share similar experiences, such as grief, loss, trauma, or specific medical conditions (e.g., cancer survivors, transplant recipients). Examples include survivor groups, veterans groups, PTSD groups, grief support groups, and abuse support groups.

• **Faith-Based Support Systems:** These systems offer spiritual guidance, community, and support through prayer, prayer groups, meditation groups, and other faith-based practices.

• **Pastoral Care:** Many organizations, including hospice and other healthcare providers, offer pastoral care services to provide spiritual and emotional support.

• **Social Workers:** Social workers can provide a range of support services, including counseling, resource referrals, and advocacy.

Mindfulness can be a valuable complement to these other forms of support. It can help you:

• **Become more aware of your emotions and thoughts:** Mindfulness techniques can help you identify and understand your emotional responses to grief, loss, or transitions.

• **Develop coping skills:** Mindfulness can teach you techniques for managing difficult emotions and reducing stress.

• **Cultivate self-compassion:** Mindfulness can help you treat yourself with kindness and understanding during challenging times.

- **Enhance the therapeutic process:** Mindfulness can deepen your awareness during therapy sessions, allowing you to engage more fully with the process.

By integrating mindfulness with other forms of support, you can create a comprehensive and holistic approach to healing and well-being.

In-Depth Content Completed:

Next, we explore the "success stories," present the chapter conclusion, and present the various exercises and visualizations for this chapter.

VI. Examples and Success Stories:

The following anonymized examples illustrate how mindfulness techniques have supported individuals in navigating various forms of grief, loss, and life transitions. While each person's experience is unique, these stories highlight the potential of mindfulness to cultivate greater self-awareness, acceptance, and resilience during challenging times.

Example 1: Navigating the Loss of a Loved One: Sarah (name changed) experienced profound grief after the sudden loss of her spouse. She found it difficult to concentrate, sleep, or experience any joy. In addition to seeking support from a grief counselor, a skilled medical massage practitioner, family and friends, Sarah began to incorporate mindfulness tools, particularly mindful breathing and mindful body scans. Through these approaches, Sarah began to notice the physical sensations associated with her grief, including a muscular tightness in her chest, trouble with digestion, and other areas of tension, discomfort, and strain. By gently acknowledging these sensations without bias or rejection, she found that these sensations, in combination with her other support systems, gradually began to lessen in intensity. Mindfulness also helped her to become more aware of her thoughts, thought patterns and self-talk, allowing her to observe and embrace her grief without getting carried away by rumination or upheavals. Over time, mindfulness, in conjunction with professional counseling, helped Sarah navigate her grief journey with greater self-compassion, improved self-care, and a new-found appreciation of her spouse, and acceptance of the new life that was ahead.

Example 2: Coping with a Major Life Transition: David (name changed) faced significant anxiety and uncertainty after a major unexpected career change. He found himself constantly worrying about the future and finances, and struggled to adapt to his job loss, and even his new job situation. Initially, between the time the old job ended, and the new one began, David first connected with a career counselor, significantly increased his networking time, began to exercise more and spend more time in nature, and also adopted some basic mindfulness techniques, focusing primarily on breathwork and mindful movement during his nature excursions. Through this multi-prong approach, David began to embrace new-found skills and techniques that helped him focus on the task at hand rather than getting lost in his fears and anxieties about the future, which allowed him to create dedicated times where he could plan the next steps of his career path. Eventually, David also began to incorporate short timed micro-mindfulness breaks throughout his day, which not only helped him keep his stress he was also able to enjoy a less frantic action-oriented perspective in his new role.

Example 3: Managing Chronic Pain During Grief: Maria (name changed) experienced a new "out of the blue" persistent low-grade pain, that came on during her grieving period after the loss of her mother. To address both her grief and her pain, Maria began working with a therapist, was medically evaluated by her doctor to rule out any major problems, joined a local grief support group, and through a church program, was introduced to foundational mindfulness techniques, of which Maria found the mindful body scans with deep relaxation techniques, and short mindful movement exercises to be very helpful. These mindfulness tools helped Maria to become more aware of the various elements of tension she was carrying, and her suppressed feelings of grief she buried in an effort to support other family members during her mother's passing, all contributing to her chronic discomfort. Through Maria's combined efforts and approaches, she was able to effectively to not only manage her pain, but in time lessen it's impact on her life, and also cultivating an expanded self-care approach that included self-compassion and greater awareness of her inner emotional and thought-habits.

VII. Chapter 9 Exercises:

Mindfulness Techniques and Visualization Exercises for Navigating Challenging Times

Navigating challenging experiences such as grief, loss, and significant life changes can be profoundly trying, often leaving us feeling overwhelmed by a range of deeply bewildering emotions.

While there is no single "cure" for these unsettling times, mindfulness techniques and related visualization exercises offer gentle tools and strategies for navigating these experiences with greater emotional ease, mental flexibility, grace, acceptance, and strength.

The following techniques and exercises can help us connect with our present moment, cultivate a gentle self-compassion, and reveal moments of peace amidst any emotional upset.

More specifically, these techniques can help you to:

- Become more aware of your thoughts and feelings
- Manage difficult emotions
- Reduce stress and promote relaxation
- Develop greater self-compassion and acceptance
- Enhance your ability to cope with change

Exercise 1: Mindful Calming Breathing

When emotions arise related to loss or life transitions, the breath can serve as a simply yet powerful anchor to the present moment. By focusing with gentle intention on the sensations of each inhale and exhale, we are allowing any feelings of distress to simply "be," rising and falling like our breath. This doesn't mean "the feelings will go away," or we're trying to avoid our feelings; rather, we're creating a safe and buffered distance that allows us to "notice" without entanglement, in time, giving rise to a calmer clarity, non-agenda acceptance, while creating the fertile ground of personal transformation.

To engage mindful breathing awareness:

- **Find a comfortable position** that works for you, sitting, standing, leaning, or lying down.

- **Close your eyes gently,** or soften your gaze if you choose to have your eyes open.

- **Allow your awareness to settle** on your breath

- **Notice** the natural rise and fall of your chest or abdomen, and heave of the shoulders, any contractions in the neck or throat, and passing of air over your lips or through your nostrils, or any other tension or sensations you feel.

- **There's no need to change your breath** in any way; simply observe it as you follow the easy rhythm of your breath.

- **When your mind wanders**, gently allow your attention to return back to the breath.

- **Return to your surroundings** when you are ready

Even a few breaths or a few minutes of mindful breathing like this can provide a sense of calm and grounding when strong emotions arrive—breathing is our portable anchor, a tool available to us wherever and whenever we feel strong emotions arise.

Exercise 2: Mindful Body Awareness

Strong emotions can often manifest physically as tension, aches, or other discomforts in the body. This mindful body awareness exercise can help you connect with these physical sensations and release that tension. This exercise involves systematically bringing awareness to different parts of your body, noticing any sensations without judgment or the need to change anything (unless shifting your position helps ease pain or discomfort). This can be especially helpful for releasing both new and long-held tension related to emotional distress, particularly the distress that often accompanies personal loss and significant life changes.

To engage mindful body awareness:

• **Lie on your back** on a comfortable surface using a yoga pad on the floor, couch, a blanket on the grass, or even a bed (or you can sit if that's more comfortable).

• **Gently close your eyes.**

• **Starting at your feet**, bring your awareness to your toes, noticing any sensations present.

• **Then, pausing at each area**, slowly begin to move your awareness through your feet, ankles, legs, torso, arms, shoulders, neck, and head, focusing on one area at a time, pause with at least one full breath for each area.

• **As your awareness shifts** from body area to body area, simply notice any sensations without trying to change them (unless a shift in position is needed to relieve pain or discomfort).

• **If your mind wanders**, gently bring it back to the area you're focusing on and continue with your body scan until you finish with your face and head.

• **Return to your surroundings** when you are ready

This exercise is adaptable to many situations. You can try an abbreviated version while standing in line, waiting for food, or even at the theater. Don't get bogged down by the idea that you must be at home in bed, on the floor, or in a chair to do this exercise—it's your exercise, so use it when you need it and modify it to suit your needs!

This exercise can also be performed as a deep relaxation exercise, where you lay in a position that is comfortable, with knee and head supports and a blanket as needed for warmth. As you focus on each area, release any tension you find with using your breath. Continue as long as you feel benefit and are able to stay awake. This technique, is often best used as a Guided Meditation.

Exercise 3: Mindful Awareness of Emotions

As we have noted, during times of significant life changes and any associated emotional upheaval, a wide range of feelings can arise including; sadness, anger, confusion, fear, and more. Mindfulness is a tool that can support it in meeting these emotions in a new way—observing them without bias or agenda, allowing them the full experience, whether the emotions arise, endure, or fade away. This exercise is about the simple acknowledgment of emotions and all the sensations that come along with them. We simply rest in awareness, "feeling the emotions," acknowledging them, but without getting carried away by them.

To engage mindful awareness of emotions:

• **When you notice a strong or destabilizing emotion arising,** pause and take a several slow mindful breaths, either with some depth, or simply with your own comfortable natural breathing pattern. *(There are many techniques available for engaging the breath as you engage your emotions, including deep nostril inhalations combined with forceful pursed lip exhalations, and many other approaches and breathing patterns)*

• **Then, gently guide your attention toward the emotion,** the places where you feel it, noticing its different physical sensations, its intensity, how the feeling and sensations change (if they do), and any associated thoughts that arise.

• **Observe the emotion**(s) as if you were a detached observer or a friend watching someone dear, and with without trying to change any feeling or push it away, simply observe and allow the emotion to be present, understanding that it will eventually shift and pass.

• **If possible, continue this exercise**, maintaining your breath and mindful awareness, **until the intensity of the emotion begins to lessen.**

Visualization Exercises:

Exercise 4: Sending Kindness Visualization (aka, Loving-Kindness Meditation):

This visualization involves cultivating feelings of warmth, kindness, and compassion, first toward oneself and then extending those same feelings to others. This technique can be particularly helpful during times of emotional distress, when we may be struggling with self-criticism or feeling disconnected from others. It can sometimes be challenging to extend these feelings to everyone, especially those we find difficult or "annoying," or those who hold different beliefs than our own. If you find yourself struggling with this, it's perfectly okay to start small, and only visualize sending kindness to your self, and the extending the practice to your closest family and friends. In time, if you are comfortable doing so, you can extend the "sending kindness" to anything or anyone without limit.

Sending Kindness Visualization Instructions:

First, find a comfortable and safe location and get settled in a position that you can rest in for several minutes. Close your eyes gently, then...

• **Begin with yourself:** First, take a mindful breath or several breaths in whatever way is comfortable and grounding for you. Once you are feeling centered, calm, and grounded, begin to direct feelings of loving-kindness toward yourself. If you find it helpful, you can repeat phrases such as "May I be filled with loving-kindness. May I be well. May I be peaceful and at ease. May I be happy."

• **Extend to loved ones:** Then, extend these feelings to someone you feel close to, such as a family member, friend, or pet. Visualize them and repeat the same phrases, substituting "they" or their name for "I" like this: "May you be filled with loving-kindness. May you be well. May you be peaceful and at ease. May you be happy." As you send kindness outward, you may also notice a sense of warmth and well-being either rising in you or returning to you.

• **Expand gradually:** As you become more comfortable, gradually expand your circle to include a neutral person (someone you see regularly but don't know well), then to someone you find difficult, and finally to all beings. As you cultivate these feelings of loving-kindness, you may find it helpful to reflect on moments of joy and gratitude in your own life (which we touch on in Chapter 10,). This can help to amplify these positive feelings and make them more readily available to share with others.

• **When your mind wanders:** If you notice your mind wandering, simply pause and take a few mindful breaths, then gently return to the visualization where you left off, or restart if you prefer, without judgment or striving— simply relax and return to the visualization.

• **Return to your surroundings** when you are ready

Exercise 5: Sending Compassion and Relief Visualization (a modified Tonglen):

This visualization focuses specifically on sending compassion and relief to those who you recognize to be suffering. It is inspired by the traditional Tonglen practice, which involves visualizing taking on the suffering of others and sending them relief. However, in this adapted version, we focus primarily on sending compassion and relief, as the act of taking on suffering can be difficult for some people, especially those facing their own sets of difficult life challenges.

Sending Compassion and Relief Visualization Instruction:

- **First, find a comfortable and safe location** and get settled in a position that you can rest in for several minutes. Close your eyes gently, then....

- **Begin with a few mindful breaths:** First, take a mindful breath or several breaths in whatever way is comfortable, calming, and grounding for you. Once you are feeling centered and ease, proceed to the next step.

- **Visualize someone who is suffering:** Visualize someone who is suffering (someone you know personally and care about is a great place to start). It could be someone experiencing a similar loss or grief to what you are going through, or someone with an unrelated life challenge that is having a hard time.

- **On the out-breath, visualize sending them relief:** On the out-breath, visualize sending them soothing relief in the form of light, warmth, healing energy, or feelings of peace and well-being. You can imagine this as a gentle stream of light flowing from your heart to theirs, or from your eyes, forehead, face or mouth. The color of the light is up to you. Just work with what feels natural for you.

- **As you become more comfortable:** You can extend this visualization to include other people who are suffering, including families you know, or entire communities suffering a catastrophic event, or even entire countries experience strife, and eventually extending to all living beings.

- **When your mind wanders:** If you notice your mind wandering, simply pause and take a few mindful breaths, then gently return to the visualization where you left off, or restart if you prefer, without judgment or striving— simply relax and return to the visualization.

- **Return to your surroundings** when you are ready.

Mindful Movement Exercises

Mindful Walking:

Why Mindful Walking and How it Can Help:
Mindful walking can be particularly helpful when you feel restless, agitated, or overwhelmed by thoughts. It can help you ground yourself in the present moment and connect with the world around you. This can be especially helpful when navigating loss or changes in environment or routine.

Mindful Walking Exercise:

• Find a quiet place where you can walk without distractions.

• Pay attention to the sensation of your feet making contact with the ground.

• Notice the movement of your body as you walk.

• Pay attention to the sights, sounds, and smells around you.

• If your mind wanders, gently redirect your attention back to the present moment.

• Continue this exercise for 10-15 minutes.

Mindful Nature Walks:

Why Mindful Nature Walks and How it Can Help:
Connecting with nature can be incredibly grounding and restorative during times of change. Mindful nature walks engage all your senses, helping you to connect with the present moment and find peace in the natural world.

Mindful Nature Walks Exercise:

• Find a natural setting where you can walk without distractions.

• Pay attention to the sights, sounds, smells, and textures around you.

• Notice the movement of your body as you walk, feeling your feet making contact with the ground.

• Allow yourself to be fully present in the natural environment.

More Helpful Exercises: One

Mindful Reflection:

Why Mindful Reflection, and How it Can Help:

Reflecting on your experiences, values, and sources of meaning can help you find a sense of purpose and direction during times of transition. This exercise can be especially helpful in making sense of loss and finding new meaning in life.

Mindful Reflection Exercise:

- Find a quiet place to sit or lie down.

- Reflect on your values, what is truly important to you.

- Consider how your current situation aligns with those values.

- Reflect on any lessons you have learned from past experiences.

More Helpful Exercises: Two

Finding Meaning In Loss Exercise:

Why Finding Meaning In Loss Exercise, and How it Can Help: Finding meaning in loss is a crucial part of the healing process. This exercise encourages reflection on the lessons learned and the potential for personal growth that can emerge from difficult experiences.

Finding Meaning In Loss Exercise:

- Reflect on the loss or transition you have experienced.

- Consider what you have learned from this experience.

- Identify any ways in which you have grown or changed as a result.

- Consider how this experience might shape your future.

For additional support in navigating difficult emotions and transitions, you may also find helpful visualization exercises that were covered in Chapter 6: Visualization: Another Layer of Mindfulness.

More Helpful Exercises: Three

RAIN Technique for Emotional Processing:

Why the RAIN Technique, and How it Can Help:
The RAIN technique is especially useful for processing difficult emotions that arise during loss and transition. It provides a structured way to acknowledge, allow, investigate, and nurture your emotions, promoting self-compassion and healing.

RAIN Technique Exercise:

• **Recognize:** Acknowledge and name the emotion you are experiencing (e.g., "sadness," "anger," "fear").

• **Allow:** Allow the emotion to be there without trying to push it away or judge it.

• **Investigate:** Gently investigate the physical sensations associated with the emotion (e.g., tightness in the chest, stomach ache).

• **Nurture:** Respond to the emotion with kindness and compassion, as you would to a friend who is suffering.

More Helpful Exercises: Four

Self-Compassion Break:

Why the Self-Compassion Break, and How it Can Help: During times of loss and transition, it's easy to be hard on ourselves, judging our reactions and feeling inadequate. The self-compassion break provides a way to offer ourselves kindness and understanding, just as we would to a friend going through a difficult time.

Self-Compassion Break Exercise:

- Think of a situation in your life that is causing you stress or pain.

- Say to yourself, "This is a moment of suffering."

- Acknowledge that suffering is a part of the human experience: "Suffering is a part of life."

- Put your hands over your heart or another comforting place on your body.

- Say to yourself, "May I be kind to myself in this moment."

More Helpful Exercises: Five

Gratitude Technique:

Why Gratitude Techniques, and How it Can Help:
Even during times of loss and transition, there are often
things to be grateful for. Cultivating gratitude can help shift
your focus from what you've lost to what you still have,
fostering resilience and hope.

Gratitude Exercise:

• Take a few moments to reflect on things you are grateful
for, no matter how small.

• Consider things like your health, your relationships,
your home, or simple pleasures like a warm cup of tea.

• You can write down your gratitudes in a journal or
simply reflect on them mentally.

Five Gentle End-of-Life Exercises

Finding Comfort & Ease:

During that period of time when our days and hours are slipping away, and while we are still aware and coherent, the basic mindfulness tools we have outlined in other chapters—mindful breathing and body awareness—can still be used to help ease anxiety, worry, fear, and other emotions, as well as assisting us to relax into our end-of-life process with a degree of comfort and ease.

We believe some of the most effective tools that can be incorporated into the end-of-life process focus on relaxing sensory experiences, positive memories, positive visualizations, as well as gentle ambient support techniques. The following list is offered as gentle invitations to support you during this transitional time. There is no right or wrong way to engage with them; choose what resonates most and adapt them as needed.

For more detailed guidance on these and other supportive techniques, please refer to:

- One Breath, Chapter 3, Page 57
- Just 10 Breaths, Chapter 4, Page 80
- Breath & Body Awareness, This Chapter, Page 269, 270
- Cultivating Gratitude, See Previous Page 284
- Visualizations & Other Exercises, see following pages

Exercise One for the End-of-Life Journey

Guided Imagery/Nature Visualization:

Why Guided Imagery/Nature Visualizations, and How They Can Support Relaxation and Inner Peace: Guided imagery and nature visualizations offer a gentle and comforting peace and tranquility. By engaging our senses and imagining peaceful settings, we can create a sense of calm and ease within ourselves, which can be particularly helpful during times of stress or discomfort.

Exercise: Imagine yourself in a peaceful natural setting and imaging that all your senses are fully engaged. Perhaps you are in a quiet forest, surrounded by your favorite tall trees with the soft sounds of birdsong and the rustling of leaves. Feel the gentle breeze on your skin and the soft earth beneath your feet and the warm sun on your face. Breathe in the fresh, earthy scent of the forest. Or perhaps you are on a tranquil beach, listening to the rhythmic crashing of waves, feeling the warm sun on your skin and the cool sand beneath your toes. Smell the cool salty air and feel the gentle breeze on your face. Allow yourself to fully immerse in your peaceful scene, letting go of any tension or worries.

Alternative Option: We encourage readers to use headphones to listen to any "Guided Nature Meditations" audio files they like (online or as downloads) as an easy way to reap the benefits of this deep relaxation tool.

Exercise Two for the End-of-Life Journey

Positive Memory Recall:

Why Positive Memory Recall, and How It Can Allow for Positive Emotions: Recalling positive memories can bring a sense of joy, comfort, and connection to the past. By revisiting cherished moments, we can experience the positive emotions associated with them, offering a gentle respite from challenging emotions or any bodily discomfort.

Exercise: Bring to mind a cherished memory—a time when you felt joy, love, or deep contentment. Allow yourself to fully immerse in the memory, noticing the sights, sounds, smells, and emotions associated with it. Relive the experience as vividly as possible, savoring the positive feelings it evokes. Take your time and savor this moment of reconnection.

Additional Suggestion: Consider writing down the details of this memory, focusing on the sensory details and emotions. This can create a tangible reminder of positive experiences.

Exercise Three for the End-of-Life Journey

Deep Relaxation/Release:

Why Deep Relaxation/Release, and How It Can Support Relaxation and Inner Peace: Deep relaxation and release techniques can help to ease physical tension and promote a sense of calm within the body. By gently releasing areas of tightness or discomfort, we can create space for greater ease and relaxation.

Exercise: Gently bring your awareness to your body. Notice any areas of tension or tightness. As you do, you may find it helpful to gently bring your awareness to your breath, as described in Chapters 3 and 4. Without judgment, simply allow those areas to soften and release, letting go of any holding or resistance.

Additional Suggestion: If you find it difficult to identify areas of tension, try gently tensing and then releasing different muscle groups in your body. This can help you become more aware of where you hold tension.

Exercise Four for the End-of-Life Journey

Light Visualization:

Why Light Visualization, and How It Can Support Relaxation and Inner Peace: Visualizing a gentle, warm light can create a sense of peace, comfort, and connection. This exercise can be especially helpful in fostering a sense of calm, comfort, ease, and well-being.

Exercise: Imagine a warm, gentle white light filling your body, starting from your toes and gradually spreading upwards to the top of your head. Feel this light radiating outwards, encompassing all beings and all things with a sense of peace and loving-kindness. As you visualize this light, you may find it helpful to connect with your breath, as discussed in Chapters 3 and 4, allowing each breath to deepen your sense of peace and an expanded experience of loving-kindness.

Alternative Approach: Some people find it helpful to visualize a color other than white, such as a soft blue, green, or gold. Experiment with different colors and see what resonates with you.

Exercise Five for the End-of-Life Journey

Music and Aromatherapy— Resting in their Soothing Ambiance:

Why and How Music and Aromatherapy Can Support Deep Relaxation: Music and aromatherapy can provide a gentle and soothing sensory experience, creating a relaxing and comforting atmosphere. These tools can help to ease tension, promote deep relaxation, and foster and support a sense of contentment, ease, and well-being.

Exercise: You may find comfort in listening to music that soothes and uplifts you. Explore different genres and find what brings you a sense of peace. Similarly, gentle aromas may enhance your sense of well-being.

Additional Suggestion: Consider creating a dedicated "relaxation space" where you can listen to music or use aromatherapy.

(Note: It's important to be mindful of scent sensitivities in yourself and others, including family members, caregivers, or healthcare providers. Additionally, aromatherapy may be contraindicated in some medical settings or treatments. Please consult with your healthcare provider or other appropriate medical professional before using aromatherapy.)

VIII. Chapter 9 Conclusion:

Together in this long chapter, we looked at how mindfulness can be a valuable support tool during the emotionally challenging times surrounding our experiences with grief and loss, as well as major life changes. We've explored how simple techniques like mindful breathing, tuning into your body, and really noticing what's around you can help you ride the waves of these difficult emotions, manage many of the physical discomforts we might be feeling, while creating an opening for some peace of mind, self-compassion, and a more receptive approach amidst the upheaval. We also touched on the importantance of reaching out for support—whether it's talking to a counselor, joining a support group, or connecting with other resources in your community.

It's so important to remember that there's no "right" way to go through grief, loss, or any major life change. Be kind to yourself during these times. Embrace self-compassion—acknowledging the pain and the struggles, all without judging yourself for feeling the way you do. And please remember that asking for help, whether from a trusted friend, a family member, or another support system, is a sign of self-care and strength, not weakness. We all need a little support sometimes, and learning how to be okay with asking for help when you feel the need is a valuable skill.

And while going through grief and loss can be incredibly difficult, it can also be a time of deep gratitude, powerful growth and important positive change. If we see mindfulness as a reliable tool in our arsenal for meeting life's challenges, it can be a truly supportive companion during our most challenging times, helping us tap into our own inner calm, even when things are upsetting and feel really tough.

By learning to be more aware of what's happening inside our minds, our emotions, and our bodies, as well as the world around us, while stepping into a gentler acceptance of situations as they are, and treating ourselves and others with kindness, we can navigate life's big shifts and challenges with a little more poise, self-confidence, and ease, while seeing that hope can rise once again.

IX. Looking Ahead to Chapter 10: Bringing Mindfulness into Your Life

And finally we head into the final chapter where I will review the core principles we have covered, lightly touch on **Mindfulness In Relationships**, and **Mindfulness and Senior Safety**. We will also present ways **Integrate Mindfulness into Daily Life** and how to **Sustain and Expand Your Mindfulness Journey**, followed by words of encouragement and some closing thoughts.

Chapter 10

"Let the beauty of what you love
be what you do."

Rumi

"The key is not to block out all the noise,
but to learn to listen to it differently."

Mingyur Rinpoche

"When everything seems to be going
against you, remember that the airplane
takes off against the wind, not with it."

Henry Ford

CHAPTER LEVEL TABLE OF CONTENTS

Chapter 10 : Bringing Mindfulness into Your Life

Chapter 10

Bringing Mindfulness into Your Life

I. Introduction:

The potential benefits of mindfulness for seniors are vast. Even in the face of significant life challenges, emotional upheaval, and physical hardships, mindfulness offers us the opportunity to experience and embody a kinder and compassionate open approach to all of life, unburdened from the mental and emotional confines we have created and clung to.

In this final chapter, I will review ways to bring mindfulness into your daily routines, including new tips for recognizing and working with difficult emotions and life challenges, and will revisit the idea about how savoring and enjoying life is as important as working with its upsets, and introduce new areas where mindfulness can be applied. And then I'll conclude with some encouragement, next steps for those interested, and perhaps most importantly, revisit how even simple mindfulness engagements can transform your life.

I see this chapter as your mindfulness-life bridge, connecting core principles and techniques to your everyday world, while offering guidance for cultivating a sustainable, comfortable, and personally appropriate long-term engagement with mindfulness, at a pace and level that feels right for you.

Revisiting Our Core Mindfulness Principles

Before we explore new applications of mindfulness, let's briefly review the three core principles that underpin many mindfulness approaches. These are: awareness, kindness/ acceptance, and curiosity.

As a reminder, our approach is slightly different, using phrasing that reflects our subtly different, yet complementary approach, which has been overlaid on traditional mindfulness foundations. Here is a recap of those:

- Instead of traditional non-judgment, I encourage a non-biased, non-agenda, 'embracing and allowing'.

- I suggest 'revealing' inherent wisdom rather than 'seeking'.

- There is encouragement for 'effortless being' instead of practice-oriented approaches.

- The idea of 'inherent wholeness' beyond perceived imperfections is presented.

The information presented in this book has been envisioned to be as easy and flexible as possible, and it is my hope that it has delivered a wisdom-driven perspective that embodies a relaxed approach that allows you to settle into clear unbiased gentle awareness.

• I think of our approach as life-centric, not practice-centric, without the requirement of formal meditation, though we certainly do not discourage meditation adoption if you are so inclined.

• It is my belief that by understanding these very subtle distinctions, you will be able to more easily integrate mindfulness in a personalized way that aligns with your unique needs.

II. Integrating Mindfulness into Daily Life

As you know, I am all about bringing mindfulness to whatever life throws at us, whenever and wherever, and encourage an as-needed, on-demand approach tailored to your inclinations and needs. In this section, I will revisit a few ways we have already touched on and explore additional ways that you can easily weave mindfulness into various aspects of your daily routine, allowing you to meet life head-on, transforming ordinary moments into opportunities for healing, transformation, and connection.

Mindful Mornings

We already touched on one aspect of this in Mindful Morning Beverage (see page 86). Begin your day with intention and awareness. Here are some other ways you can try or play with some "micro-morning-mindfulness" approaches:

• When you first wake up, allow yourself to rest for a few moments in bed, becoming aware of your surroundings, your breath, your body sensations. Take a few mindful breaths. Continue mindfully as you rise and begin your morning routines.

• Take a moment to step outside and notice and appreciate the dawn or morning. Step into the morning cool. Take a few mindful breaths, enjoying the start of a new day.

• Before moving into the main part of your day, either before starting those tasks or when getting into a car or moving to the next location for the next activity, pause and take a mindful breath or two before continuing. Continue with mindful breaths as you travel and upon arrival, if desired.

Mindfulness at Work/During Activities

No matter if you are engaged in work, hobbies, daily tasks, or simple pleasures, to the degree you are able, keep the jewel of your mindfulness (as we discussed in Chapter 5) at the ready... It's a great addition to enrich your day. As your day moves along, no matter if you are facing a difficult situation, and arduous task, or simply enjoying a stroll or a round of golf, taking a few mindful breaths and an intentional pause during the course of your day as needed or as inclined, can be a wonderful way to help enrich the day's activities, keep you calm, and even help focus, creativity and enhance your day's enjoyment. Engaging with mindfulness, even in small ways and at your own pace, can transform your life into something savored and remarkable.

Mindful Evenings

As the day winds down, take a few mindful moments to settle into the close of your day. Reflect on the day's ebb and flow, taking a few mindful breaths to release its hold. Settle into your evening routine, savoring your meal and those you share your life with. Intentionally embrace the evening's routines, and when settling into your restful sleep, another mindful breath or two, with a quick body scan and tension release can support a rejuvenating night's rest for your mind and body.

Emotional Upset

If you begin to notice some emotional upset, to the degree you are able, pause (and if needed, step away from the source of the upset), take one or more mindful breaths, allowing the tension and upset to fade. Continue with your breath until you feel you have regained your emotional equilibrium. *(Often referred to as the "STOP Technique": Use the STOP technique to manage stress: **Stop** what you are doing, **Take** a breath, **Observe** your thoughts, feelings, and sensations, and **Proceed** with intention)*

Mental Agitation

During the course of a day, it is not uncommon to feel times of frustration, complaining, or blaming. When you notice your mind getting agitated in any way, pause (and if needed, step away from the source of the agitation), take one or more mindful breaths, allowing the agitation and upset to fade. Continue with your breath until you feel you have regained your mental balance.

Happiness & Joy

There are many opportunities each day to simply notice and enjoy the world around you. When you feel a sense of appreciation, gratitude, encounter beauty, see or receive a kindness from another person, or are spending time in activities you enjoy, or having experiences with people you cherish, pause and take one or more mindful breaths, allowing the awe and appreciation to flow into you. Continue with your breath and expansive sense of appreciation until you feel joyously fulfilled.

By incorporating just a few of the previous simple mindfulness techniques into your daily routine you cam **reset** your internal state, **reorient** your intentions, and **recenter** your relationship with the world.

III. Mindfulness & Relationships

Relationships are the threads that infuse, weave, and color the rich tapestry of our lives, reflecting our connections to the people and world around us. From the intimate bonds we share with family, close friends, and life partners, to the social connections within our communities, the functional relationships with caregivers and service providers, and even the people just passing by in our peripheral view, we are all interacting and connecting in many important ways, some quite subtle and others much more apparent.

These connections, whether deep or fleeting, contribute to our feeling of belonging and well-being as well as shaping our sense of self. By recognizing the far-reaching implications of how relationships shape our world, we can deepen these connections and enhance richness, enjoyment, and our overall quality of life by intentionally approaching relationships with mindful sensitivity, at a level that feels right for you.

A Note On The Subtle Aspects of Negative Self-Talk and Mindful Relationships

The subtle interactions we have with others aren't limited to external exchanges; they also include the internal dialogues we have with ourselves, and the way we think about, refer to, assess, and judge others, which can significantly shape our internal mental and emotional landscape, and profoundly influence our relationships with others and ourselves. As traditions like Buddhism, Hinduism, Christianity, Islam, and Judaism teach, 'harsh speech' extends beyond spoken words to encompass negative thoughts and judgments, which create internal barriers to mindful connection.

These internal dialogues, often operating beneath our conscious awareness, can subtly sabotage our attempts at mindful connection, creating biases and agendas that hinder genuine understanding. This is where the practice of non-bias/no-agenda listening becomes crucial, allowing the internal dialogues to naturally subside, allowing us to approach relationships with greater receptivity, openness and clarity. For instance, if we're constantly judging a family member's behavior, it's difficult to truly listen to them with an open heart. Or if we're blaming a caregiver for our frustrations, we may miss opportunities for genuine connection.

When you notice these kinds of internal dialogues (blaming, criticizing, belittling, etc), ask yourself:

• *Who is it that has the bias or agenda that is pervading these thoughts and self-talk and what is the purpose of these harsh thoughts?*

Here is how we can think of mindful relationships:

First on the list is the ideas of an open and receptive no-agenda, non-bias mental and emotional stance when interacting with others. This is an expansion of the "present-moment awareness" concept, but placed into the context of relationships. We acknowledge this may not be easy... but from my perspective the challenge is worth a try.

You have probably heard of these "relationship guidelines;" *active listening, empathy, kindness, compassion, and respect for boundaries.* But we shift those approaches slightly like this:

- **Active listening becomes "receptive open-hearted, non-bias, no-agenda listening"**

- **Empathy, kindness, and compassion, rather than something that is "performed" or cultivated, it is something that naturally arises with the "receptive open-hearted non-bias, no-agenda listening"** (as referenced in the first bullet point)

- **The naturally arising qualities mentioned above equally apply to "respect for boundaries."**

A mindful approach to relationships allows us to truly connect with others and supports the natural and inherent wholeness present in everyone to unfold.

In my view, the gentle cultivation of mindful relationships is not about forced effort and adhering to preconceived notions of what a "mindful relationship should be", but rather an effortless flow that allows natural expression to emerge. In the following sections, we will explore practical ways to experience mindful connections and relationships in your life.

Additional Relationship Ideas to Consider

Building upon the foundation of mindful relationships, there are several additional facets to reflect on that can impact your connections and sense of well-being, either positively or negatively. These ideas address common challenges and opportunities, offering practical ways to integrate mindfulness into various relationship dynamics. By exploring these areas, you can deepen your understanding of how mindfulness can support you in navigating the ever-evolving landscape of relationships.

Loneliness and Isolation:

The Challenge: Loneliness and isolation can create feelings of disconnection and emotional distress, particularly for seniors who may experience reduced social interaction.

The Opportunity *(and benefit)*: Even if your external connections are limited, mindfulness offers an opportunity to cultivate a deeper connection with yourself and enrich the relationships you do have. Deepening your engagement with the present moment can result in improved life contentment and ease.

The Mindfulness Approach: By opening and relaxing into the present fullness of life, engaging and exploring your senses and surroundings, and deeply engaging with the relationships available to you can minimize the impacts of loneliness. For example, engaging in mindful activities like gardening, listening to your favorite music, or simply savoring a favorite food or comforting warm beverage can help you feel more grounded and at ease. Adding depth to your life experiences helps many seniors to reduce feelings of isolation.

Relationship Changes and Loss *(See Chapter 9)*:

The Challenge: Seniors often experience changes in relationships due to loss, illness, or relocation, which can lead to feelings of grief, uncertainty, and emotional distress. These transitions, while a natural part of life, can trigger a wide range of powerful and unsettling emotions.

The Opportunity *(and benefit)*: Mindfulness can provide a sense of grounding and resilience during these times of change, allowing you to meet the challenges with increased ease and emotional stability while supporting and honoring the memories and helping you retain your sense of comfort and continuity.

The Mindfulness Approach: When experiencing loss or relationship shifts that are unsettling, working with mindful, non-biased, open acceptance of your emotions can be a helpful approach. Allow yourself time to adjust to the changes and grieve or mourn the losses as needed. Reflecting on the loss while also continuing to engage in activities that bring you comfort and connection to other aspects of your life can be very helpful as well.

For example, mindful journaling, gentle walks in nature, or sharing memories with loved ones can help you process emotions and regain your sense of natural ease and grace.

Remember, these emotional challenges are a universally human experience, and strong emotions around change and loss can be significant, and the experiences and expressions of them is always a deeply personal journey.

The Two Faces of Compassion in Relationships:

The Challenge: Relationships can be challenging, and it's easy to fall into patterns of criticism and judgment towards yourself and others.

When frustration or tempers are running hot, we may find ourselves being overly harsh on ourselves for the mistakes or shortcomings we perceive in ourselves, or conversely, we may become angry and impatient with those we care about for some behavior or perceived uncaring act. This can lead to feelings of disconnection, resentment, and emotional distress, hindering our ability to experience and relax into the harmonious and genuinely sincere connections we previously shared.

The Opportunity *(and benefit)*: Recognizing that compassion has two faces—self-compassion and compassion for others—lends a transformative perspective to relationships. Self-compassion, the approach of treating yourself with kindness, understanding, and acceptance, forms the bedrock of our compassionate connections, and without it, compassion for others cannot be revealed.

By gently nurturing authentic self-compassion (not to be confused with a self-absorbed focus), you are able to stabilize the inner resources that help you navigate relationship challenges with greater clarity and emotional resilience. This translates into genuine self-care, self-nurture, and healthy self-talk, which then naturally extends to a more nurturing and understanding attitude towards others.

Embracing and recognizing the importance of the two faces of compassion, you lay the groundwork for deeper, more authentic connections, imbued with a naturally arising empathy, patience, and sincere respect.

The Mindfulness Approach: First, I want to restate that compassion, whether for ourselves or others, from the perspective of this book, is our natural state that is always shining. It is the negative self-talk, harsh speech, and thoughts, plus the myriad mental habits, emotional patterns, and perceptual overlays we project that conceal it. So pursuing or practicing compassion is not really our approach, where instead, we gently lean into the notions of non-biased acceptance, open receptive non-agenda listening, and so on (as previously discussed throughout this book).

For some, what I have found to be helpful when you notice self-criticism arising, simply pause, mindfully take a breath or two or three, and relax into the wider spaciousness of the moment, simply being aware, allowing the waves of emotions and thoughts that rise and fall without intervention.

If you feel the need for additional support and self-care, offer yourself some words of kindness and encouragement, or remind yourself that everyone makes mistakes and that you too are worthy of your kindness.

Extend this mindful awareness to your interactions with others. When you experience conflict or frustration, remember the calming and grounding power of the breath, and when listening is required, be fully attentive without bias or agenda and allow your natural compassion, empathy, understanding, and forgiveness to naturally arise. And when it is time to speak, to the best of your ability, do so calmly, mindfully, and with care and respect. By consistently engaging with these approaches, you can shift and enrich the dynamics of your relationships and discover an authentic, fulfilling, and balanced new way to interact with others.

Digital Relationships:

The Challenge: Digital relationships are increasingly important, especially for seniors who have a need or desire to stay connected with friends, loved ones, and family. However, they can also present many challenges, such as navigating technology, encountering online scams, and managing the emotional impact of consuming overwhelming or divisive media content. In today's challenging news cycles, it is easy to see how we seniors may experience heightened anxiety and distress from both reputable and and sensationalized news reports, as well and social media feeds and the seemingly endless stream of "opinions" that are being presented... All with the potential to negatively affect our relationships and our sense of overall well-being.

Additionally, the potential for frustration and disappointment can arise from digital interactions, such as non-responses in emails, inarticulate responses that don't accurately convey the intended message, or auto-fill responses that are inaccurate, leading to feelings of disconnect and upset.

The Opportunity *(and benefit)*: By choosing to approach digital interactions mindfully, you set yourself up for successfully navigating the challenges while also reaping the many benefits that online interactions offer. Implementing a mindful media consumption approach not only allows you to be discerning about the content you consume, which has the potential benefit of significantly reducing anxiety and supporting a calmer emotional landscape, but mindful digital communication can also help you navigate the inevitable misunderstandings that arise, while mindful digital communication can also strengthen those connections you are trying to foster, even in the absence of face-to-face interaction. *(Technology resource note: If you need assistance working with technology or finding online sources that are safe for seniors, reach out to your local senior support network or contact reputable online senior support platforms such as AARP.)*

The Mindfulness Approach: Begin by setting clear intentions for your digital interactions. Before checking emails or social media, take a moment to breathe and center yourself. Practice mindful media consumption by being aware of the content you consume and how it affects you. Set boundaries for your online time and take regular breaks from screens. In your online communications, practice mindful listening and empathy. Take a moment to pause and reflect before responding to emails or social media posts. Remember to extend the same kindness and compassion to yourself and others in your digital interactions as you would in face-to-face interactions.

When encountering upsetting online content, whether from a news source, a family member, a post with hateful speech, or other offensive or upsetting content, recognize that you have the ability to "step away" *(Remember the STOP Technique: Use the STOP technique to manage stress: Stop what you are doing, Take a breath, Observe your thoughts, feelings, and sensations, and Proceed with intention).* This might mean blocking, deleting, closing the offending source, or simply getting away from the screen and shifting your activity to something more nurturing and calming.

Taking ACTION when encountering challenging online content is an overlooked aspect of mindfulness, and recognizing upsets arising from online content is an important aspect of the mindful approach to digital relationships, and maybe even the crux of it. It is equally appropriate to consume and interact with uplifting and informative online content mindfully, paying attention to your body and emotions.

Recognize when you need to take a break, and then step away from the screen and engage in other supportive or necessary activities. Timers can help.

Additional Considerations:

Furthermore, be mindful of your interactions with AI (Artificial Intelligence) systems. While AI can be a valuable resource, remember that these systems have an endurance far exceeding human capacity. Additionally, be aware of the potential for AI-generated "deep-fakes" and misinformation. Practice discernment and critical thinking when interacting with AI and consuming online content. As with all digital interactions, maintain awareness of your emotional state and take breaks as needed.

Remember that online music can be a valuable resource for calming, and relaxation. Explore different genres and create playlists that support your emotional well-being. However, be mindful of copyright and legality when accessing music. Use reputable platforms that respect artists' rights. Be aware of the volume at which you listen to music to protect your hearing health. Also, pay attention to the emotional impact of different genres and songs, choosing music that supports your well-being.

Intergenerational Relationships:

The Challenge: Intergenerational relationships, while deeply rewarding, can also present unique challenges. Differences in age, life experiences, and cultural backgrounds can lead to communication gaps and misunderstandings. Seniors may find it difficult to connect with younger generations who have different values, communication styles, and technological fluency. Conversely, younger generations may struggle to understand the perspectives and experiences of their elders. These gaps can sometimes lead to feelings of disconnection, frustration, and conflict, hindering the potential for mutually enriching relationships.

The Opportunity *(and benefit)***:** Intergenerational relationships offer a wealth of opportunities for mutual growth, learning, and connection. By approaching these relationships with mindfulness, you can bridge the gaps and cultivate deeper richer relationships with increased mutual appreciation and insight. Seniors can share their wisdom and life experiences, while younger generations can offer fresh perspectives, technological tips, and explanations.

Using mindful communication approaches we have previously outlined in some depth, can support meaningful dialogues and create a sense of shared understanding and connection. By embracing the richness of intergenerational interactions, you can build and enjoy a supportive and enriching network that benefits everyone involved.

The Mindfulness Approach: When engaging in intergenerational interactions, begin by adopting an open and receptive, no-agenda, non-biased mental and emotional stance. Allow yourself to listen calmly, with warmth, and the spirit of open-receptivity, without interrupting, allowing empathy, kindness, and compassion to naturally arise from your open-hearted approach.

Seek to understand the other person's perspective, even if it differs from your own, allowing for the natural unfolding of respect for boundaries. When it is time to communicate, express your thoughts and feelings with clarity and kindness, mindful of the calming and grounding power of the breath.

Create opportunities for shared experiences, whether in-person or online, such as family gatherings, outings, or activities that both generations enjoy, allowing the natural flow of connection to emerge. Be patient and understanding when encountering communication gaps or misunderstandings, recognizing that these are opportunities for deeper understanding and connection.

Practice mindful questioning, asking for clarification when needed and using thoughtful, relevant questions to deepen your dialogue, which can serve as a powerful and meaningful way to express your caring and meaningful connection, demonstrate your interest, and support your relationship's growth and enrichment.

Remember that intergenerational relationships are a valuable source of wisdom, support, and connection, and that by adopting this mindful approach, you are allowing the natural and inherent wholeness present in everyone to unfold.

IV. Senior Safety and Well-Being

Maintaining well-being and supporting our safety as seniors is an increasingly important consideration as we age. Mindfulness offers an effective framework of strategies and tools that can support physical and mental health, which can have a direct influence on our safety. Issues such as enhanced balance, fall prevention, and situational awareness, are all important elements of the senior safety landscape.

Crucially, some preliminary studies indicate that mindfulness may also play a role in slowing mental decline, a serious consideration with significant implications, one of which is seen in its potential for poor decision-making, resulting in significantly increased risks for serious accidents or even life-threatening decisions (such as forgetting to take medications, not recognizing or dismissing serious physical symptoms, not recognizing safety hazards at home or when out in the world, etc).

By engaging mindfulness techniques, as seniors, we are better equipped to make more informed, safe, and health-supporting choices for our physical and mental well-being, with the added benefit of enhanced life enjoyment. Integrating mindfulness into daily life allows us to meet and navigate aging with greater skill, enhanced awareness, and improved confidence.

In the following sections, we will explore practical ways to apply mindfulness to enhance our safety through these different contexts:

- **Physical Health** (including mindful hygiene techniques and its effects on sleep, nutrition, and exercise)

- **Fall Prevention and Balance** (including practical tips for mindful walking and creating a safe home environment.)

- **Situational Awareness and Safety** (including explorations of ways to enhance your awareness of the surroundings and identify safety concerns)

Mindfulness for Physical Health:

The Challenge: As seniors, we may find ourselves facing a range of physical health challenges, ranging from declining energy levels, chronic pain, decreased immune function, longer healing and recovery times, to sleep challenges, nutritional deficiencies, and even loss of mobility and bodily functions.

Those health challenges seniors face are very real and potentially very serious. And, while I encourage a mindful approach to support your health, I feel it is my responsibility to outline the potential negative ramifications when a non-mindful or too-casual approach to our health is taken in later years of life.

From my perspective, a non-mindfulness approach (ie; not considering the ramifications of our decisions), can gloss over the direct impact daily habits and choices can have on our overall well-being. This can lead to a dangerous cycle of declining health, increasing physical limitations or impairments, resulting in greater pressures on our health, while also negatively impacting our safety.

While a mindful approach can support our physical health in a variety of ways, conversely, a NON-mindful approach can further stress existing challenges, and potentially create new issues to deal with as well.

For example, ignoring physical discomfort, dismissing warning signs, or "accepting symptoms" without addressing them, can lead to delayed diagnoses and more serious health complications. Similarly, mindless eating habits can contribute to weight gain or nutritional imbalances and deficiencies, while neglecting sleep can impair cognitive function and decision-making.

Also, lapses in personal hygiene can stress and weaken the immune system. Individually or combined, these issues can negatively affect our ability to exercise and participate in the activities we enjoy while also increasing the risks of accidents and serious illness.

The Opportunity *(and benefit)*: By embracing a mindful approach to our physical health, we can not only improve our health-supporting thinking and decisions, we can directly counter the challenges that arise as we age. Where declining energy levels once hindered our daily activities, mindful approaches can revitalize us, restoring vigor and vitality. When chronic pain threatens to limit our mobility, mindfulness can offer tools to manage discomfort and enhance our range of motion.

Using mindful strategies, we can make health-supporting decisions that positively affect our immune system, reducing susceptibility to illness and promoting faster healing.

Mindful sleep techniques can help us transform restless nights into restful slumber, which can aid cognitive function, and support healthy decision-making. Also, mindful approaches to personal hygiene can support the immune system and overall physical health. Mindful eating habits can nourish our bodies, supporting and even restoring nutritional balance while supporting healthy weight management. By paying attention to our bodies' signals, we can recognize and address potential health issues early, preventing them from escalating into serious complications.

This proactive approach can break the cycle of declining health or potentially reverse it, replacing it with a journey of enhanced vitality and endurance, improved physical health and cognitive ability, while supporting and enhancing our enjoyment of life.

Mindfulness for Fall Prevention and Balance:

The Challenge: Falls are a significant health concern for seniors, with approximately one in four older adults experiencing a fall each year, according to a recent (2024) CDC study. These falls can lead to serious injuries, including hip fractures, head injuries, and even brain trauma, and are a leading cause of injury-related deaths among older adults.

Contributing factors include poor balance, physical limitations, medication side effects, vision problems, environmental hazards, and simply being unaware of your surroundings.

Even individuals who are otherwise active and capable can be prone to falls when they are not mindful of their surroundings and movements. As an example, my wife is a "full-speed ahead" sort of personality, getting things done. She freely admits that her tendency to "not pay attention" to her surroundings, has resulted in multiple falls over the years, leading to hospital visits, lost mobility, and disruptions to our lives. This underscores how a lack of mindfulness can dramatically increase the risk of falls, even for those who consider themselves steady on their feet and fully mobile.

Simply stated, we believe that a non-mindful approach to life is a significant factor that leads to increased safety risks. By "not paying attention" or allowing ourselves to get distracted or stay distracted can have serious implications including:

- Allowing us to overlook potential hazards,
- Rushing through normal activities or chores, or
- Failing to notice changes in our balance or mobility

These kinds of lapses can all contribute to our risk. In addition to the injury healing time, fear of future falls, and decreased mobility or activity resulting from the fall can ensue, all increasing the risk of more falls in the future.

The Opportunity *(and benefit)*: By cultivating mindfulness, we can significantly reduce the risk of falls and enhance our overall sense of stability and well-being. Mindful awareness allows us to become more attuned to our bodies, noticing subtle shifts in balance and potential hazards in our environment. This heightened awareness can help us make adjustments to our movements and surroundings, preventing falls before they occur.

By engaging in mindfulness techniques, we can enhance our confidence which then allows us to move with greater awareness and enhanced stability.

Furthermore, mindful movement, such as mindful walking, can strengthen our muscles, improve our coordination, and enhance our sense of movement and our body's position in relation to obstacles. Regular exercise, in conjunction with mindfulness, is particularly effective in combating the natural decline in muscle mass and bone density associated with aging, which can help mitigate common health risks. This can lead to increased stability and a reduced risk of falls.

By embracing a mindful approach, we cultivate a deeper conscious connection with our bodies, leading to improved spatial awareness, enhanced balance, and increased stability. An additional benefit that can arise is a reduced "fear of falling," which can allow us to be more active, which can then aid in reducing the risk of future falls.

The Mindfulness Approach: When it comes to fall prevention and balance, mindfulness can add a valuable contribution to safety by complementing traditional safety measures, such as non-skid surfaces, removal of tripping hazards, safety rails if needed, etc. By embracing techniques to support our present-moment awareness, we not only improve our mind/body awareness, we improve our awareness of our surroundings which translates to safer living overall as well as reduced fall risks, both at home and in travels outside of home.

Below are some mindful approaches I feel are important and beneficial for reducing fall risks, and I invite you to consider them, and potentially adopt them if they seem to be appropriate for your situation:

- **Present Moment Awareness Related to Your Body:** Cultivating awareness of bodily sensations, balance, and movement can help us notice subtle shifts and make necessary adjustments.

• **Spatial Body Awareness and Balance:** Practices such as mindful standing and mindful transitions can enhance body awareness and improve balance.

• **Mindful Walking:** Mindful walking, focusing on posture, gait, and the sensation of the ground beneath the feet, can enhance balance and stability. *(Detailed instructions for mindful walking can be found in other sections of this book.)*

• **Home Safety:** Developing a mindful perspective can be a useful aid to help you identify and then mitigate any potential fall hazards in or around your home.

Remember that mindfulness should be seen as a complementary approach to traditional fall prevention measures, including in-home exercise regimens, medical support, physical therapist-recommended exercise programs, home safety assessments, and home modifications including incorporating assistive safety devices or improving handicap access. I encourage readers to always consult with their physician, physical therapist, or health support team before engaging in any new movement or balance exercises.

Mindfulness for Situational Awareness and Safety:

The Challenge: As seniors, we often face unique challenges that can make us more vulnerable to safety risks. These risks can arise in various settings, from our own homes to public spaces and even within our social circles. Without mindful awareness, we may overlook potential hazards, misjudge situations, or fall victim to scams and exploitation.

In our homes, we might neglect to notice spoiled food, outdated medications, or tripping hazards. We may also be susceptible to exploitation by hired help or fall victim to online scams. Outside our homes, we may encounter environmental hazards, predatory individuals, or dangerous driving situations. Socially, we may struggle to recognize signs of manipulation or exploitation, even from those we consider friends.

Furthermore, factors such as cognitive decline, over-medication, or excessive alcohol consumption can impair our judgment and increase our vulnerability. Even something as simple as wearing conspicuous clothing can make us a target for unwanted attention. Additionally, non-mindful cell phone use can be a major source of distraction, affecting our situational awareness while walking, driving, or in public spaces.

These challenges highlight the need for heightened situational awareness, which can be difficult to maintain when we are distracted, stressed, or simply not paying attention. Without a strong foundation in mindfulness strategies, we may find ourselves in situations that compromise our safety and well-being.

The Opportunity *(and benefit)*: By cultivating mindfulness, we can significantly enhance our situational awareness and create a safer environment for ourselves. Mindfulness allows us to be more present and attuned to our surroundings, enabling us to recognize potential dangers before they escalate.

Through mindfulness, we can sharpen our sensory awareness, noticing subtle cues that might indicate a problem. We can also develop a stronger connection with our intuition, trusting our gut feelings when something doesn't feel right. Furthermore, mindfulness can help us maintain clear and focused thinking, avoiding cognitive biases, unfounded fears, or emotional overreactions that can lead to less-than-optimal assessments of the situation.

With increased situational awareness, we can navigate various settings with greater confidence and ease. We can identify potential hazards in our homes, recognize manipulative individuals, and make safer choices while driving or traveling. We can also minimize the impact of factors such as cognitive decline or over-medication by being more aware of our limitations and seeking appropriate support.

By integrating mindfulness into our daily lives, we can create a proactive approach to safety, empowering ourselves to make informed decisions and avoid potentially dangerous situations.

The Mindfulness Approach: Enhancing situational awareness through mindfulness involves cultivating a heightened sense of sensory awareness and attunement to your surroundings. Here are some mindful approaches to consider:

- **Mindful Observation:** Practice observing your surroundings with heightened awareness. Pay attention to details such as people's body language, potential hazards, and subtle cues that might indicate danger. For example, while waiting in your car, put down your phone, turn off the radio, and simply observe the people and activities around you, noticing their movements and potential interactions, in a "just noticing" way.

- **Regular Check-ins:** Throughout the day, practice regular "check-ins" with yourself, noticing your physical sensations, emotional state, and thought patterns. Consider incorporating regular check-ins with family, friends, or neighbors, especially when out and about alone.

- **Mindful Decision-Making:** Before making decisions, slow down and consider potential risks and consequences. Ask yourself: "What are the potential consequences of this action? Does this situation feel safe? What are my options?"

• **Trusting Intuition:** Pay attention to your gut feelings. If a situation feels uncomfortable or unsafe, trust your intuition and remove yourself from it.

• **Mindful Communication:** Practice clear and assertive communication, both verbal and non-verbal. Be aware of signs of manipulation or deception, and set healthy boundaries in your interactions.

"When in Doubt" Safety List:

• Trust your gut feeling. If a situation feels unsafe, remove yourself from it.

• Don't be afraid to ask for help. Reach out to a trusted friend, family member, or authority figure.

• Be cautious about sharing personal information with strangers.

• Avoid walking alone in poorly lit or isolated areas, especially at night.

• Be aware of your surroundings and avoid distractions, such as using your phone while walking.

• Remain aware of your physical limitations, and avoid pushing yourself beyond those limits.

By integrating these mindful approaches into your daily life, you can confidently and effectively enhance your situational awareness and create a safer environment for yourself.

V. Sustaining and Expanding Your Mindfulness Journey

Introduction:

Mindfulness is a journey that can be explored in many ways—from formal approaches and programs to casual practices—each valid and valuable. Some find comfort in setting gentle intentions and cultivating a supportive network, while others discover profound insights by simply relaxing into the open spaciousness of each moment. Neither approach is inherently 'better' than the other; they are simply different facets of the same luminous mindfulness experience. You may find yourself drawn to one more than the other, and that is perfectly fine.

If you resonate with setting intentions, remember that these are not rigid targets, but rather gentle guiding lights. Allow yourself to adjust them as needed, just as you might take a single mindful breath or ten mindful steps. Even within these intentions, there's always room to pause, to simply be, and to connect with the stillness that resides within.

And remember, there's a path that unfolds naturally, beyond our conscious plans, when we allow ourselves to simply be. Sometimes, the most profound insights arise when we release our need to control the journey. They are like the sun and the moon, both beautiful and illuminating aspects of the sky of awareness.

Regardless of the approach that speaks to you, either with a gentle nudge or even without effort or pursuit, relax into the natural caring self-kindness available and accessible at any time. Remember, there's no right or wrong way to explore mindfulness and no better or worse experience. The most important thing is to relax and release the grip of control, bias, and agenda. Stepping into the awareness that simply notices, allowing perceptions to unfold without constraint... allowing the reactions to fade into the passing stream of life, allowing natural curiosity, and compassion to arise, trusting your path and your own inner wisdom.

The Goal Approach:
Shaping Your Path & Options for Support

For those drawn to a more structured approach, setting mindful intentions can be a valuable way to guide your ongoing efforts. However, it's essential to remember that the "intentions" you establish should be both achievable and, crucially, enjoyable. From my perspective, mindfulness is, at its heart, a savoring of life's moments, of revealing joy, and relaxing and allowing the kaleidoscopic present to unfold without agenda or bias. While it's true that mindfulness can be a powerful and effective support tool for navigating life's challenges, it's the 'savor' aspect—the natural arising of appreciation, gratitude, and life satisfaction—that truly sustains our journey.

Think of it this way: if your intentions feel like burdens, or if your practice becomes a chore, a "must do" or a prescriptive task, it's unlikely you'll maintain it over the long term. Instead, consider creatively shaping intentions that spark your curiosity, ignite your enthusiasm, and beckon you to explore and enjoy the richness of your inner world and the beauty of your surroundings. Perhaps you'll intend to spend five minutes each morning simply noticing the sensations of your breath, or to take a short mindful walk in nature once a week.

The length or complexity is totally up to you! Just think in small, manageable, and enjoyable bites...like our mindful-moments exercise or the "just one bite" idea we introduced you to. Even acts with small intentions, whether to savor life or to solve a life challenge, can lead to profound shifts in your perspective and well-being.

Remember, the goal is not to become a mindless zombie, a zoned-out do-nothing person, or even to achieve some abstract state of enlightenment, but rather, to embody a deeper connection with all of life, including your inner and outer worlds.

Let your intentions be the gentle nudges and kind reminders you would get from a good friend, inviting you to relax, enjoy, and savor while meeting the present, and allowing your natural grace, ease, and joy to arise.

Identifying and utilizing support systems

While mindfulness is a solo and personal journey, being part of a supportive community or network of like-minded people can significantly enhance your mindfulness adventure.

Your support community or network could be made up of friends, family, mindfulness groups, or professionals, and also include other inspirational items such as pre-recorded guided meditations, other books, calendars or note-cards, counting stones or wrist malas, or any other expression of support that resonates with you.

VII. Exploring Mindfulness Support Options

It's important to also consider your options for supporting our mindfulness journey if you ever need a boost or want to connect to a larger community. And because finding the right support system and mindfulness approach is such a personal journey, it's important to consider many different options, and then choose what resonates with you.

Don't be afraid to adjust your approach as your needs and preferences evolve. Your mindfulness adventure is something that unfolds over time and is unique to you, so embrace the freedom to personalize it and make it your own.

Friends and Family:

Authentic and open communication about your experiences, challenges, and insights can deepen your relationships and foster mutual understanding with your supportive individuals. You can also consider engaging in some easy mindful activities together, such as taking a mindful walk in nature, sharing a mindful meal, or even enjoying a guided meditation together.

These shared experiences can create lasting memories and strengthen your bond and also help to restore your connection to your mindfulness efforts.

Mindfulness Groups (Online or In-Person):

Connecting with like-minded individuals in a mindfulness group, whether online or in person, can provide a powerful sense of community and shared learning. These groups offer a space to explore mindfulness concepts, share experiences, and learn from others on a similar journey. The shared experience can be very motivating, and provide a sense of accountability.

Participating in group meditations, discussions, and workshops can deepen your understanding of mindfulness and provide valuable insights. When you feel your mindfulness journey has drifted, slowed or needs a boost, the support and encouragement of a mindfulness group can be particularly helpful in re-engaging.

You can also consider joining our free, private, senior-only mindfulness community! (Moderated by the author)
Sign up at: mindfulness4seniors.com/join

Professional Guidance:

Seeking guidance from therapists, counselors, or mindfulness instructors can provide personalized support and expertise on your mindfulness journey. These professionals can help you navigate specific challenges, develop tailored strategies, and deepen your understanding of mindfulness principles and help you identify any underlying patterns or obstacles that may be hindering your progress.

• If you're facing difficulties with stress management, emotional regulation, or other mental health concerns, a licensed therapist or counselor can provide a safe and supportive space to explore these issues. Some therapist as skilled mindfulness teachers or practitioners and so can help you integrate a mindful approach into your daily life and develop coping mechanisms for challenging situations.

• Mindfulness instructors can offer expert guidance on various mindfulness techniques, such as meditation, breathwork, and body awareness. They can help you refine your practice, address any questions or concerns, and provide ongoing support.

Remember, seeking professional guidance or even personalized coaching support is a sign of strength and self-care. It demonstrates a commitment to your well-being and a willingness to invest in your personal growth.

Recharging and Regrounding with Nature:

Nature offers a powerful and readily accessible source of solace, renewal, and grounding. Spending time in natural environments can have a profound impact on your mindfulness practice and overall well-being.

Whether it's a walk in a park, a hike in the woods, or simply sitting by a tree, immersing yourself in nature can help you reconnect with your senses and find inner peace. The sights, sounds, and smells of nature can be a gentle reminder of the present moment, inviting you to let go of distractions and find stillness within.

When you feel your mindfulness practice has stalled or you're struggling to re-engage, nature can be a powerful ally. Its calming presence can help you release stress, clear your mind, and find a renewed sense of purpose.

Regrounding with Nature is one of our personal favorites when we need to recharge. We hope you will consider incorporating regular nature walks or outdoor mindfulness practices into your routine. Even short periods spent in nature can have a significant and beneficial impact on your well-being.

Finding Your Personal Touchstones:

Personal touchstones are sources of strength, inspiration, and recentering that can provide comfort and guidance on your mindfulness journey. They are unique to each individual and can take many forms.

Perhaps your personal touchstone is spending time in nature, feeling the sun on your skin and the earth beneath your feet. Or maybe it's your faith, finding solace and connection in prayer or meditation. It could be journaling, expressing your thoughts and feelings on paper, or engaging in another creative activity. Or simply the practice of silence, finding stillness and peace within.

Take a moment to reflect on what brings you comfort, inspiration, and a sense of grounding. What activities, places, or practices help you reconnect with yourself and find inner peace? These are your personal touchstones.

Once you've identified your touchstones, consider how you can incorporate them into your daily mindfulness practice. Perhaps you can schedule regular walks in nature, set aside time for prayer or meditation, or dedicate a few minutes each day to journaling.

By recognizing and utilizing your own personal touchstones, you can create a more fulfilling mindfulness engagement.

Inspirational Resources:

Inspirational resources can take many forms, from the wisdom of renowned mindfulness teachers to the comfort of faith-based practices.

Consider exploring the works of authors like Jon Kabat-Zinn, Pema Chödrön, or Thich Nhat Hanh for insightful perspectives on mindfulness.

For those seeking faith-based inspiration, explore resources aligned with your own beliefs. To find relevant materials, you can search for:

- '<insert your preferred faith name> + mindfulness' or
- '<insert your preferred faith name> + meditation.'

This will lead you to a wealth of periodicals, newsletters, websites, audio recordings, videos, and more. You may also find faith-centric mindfulness groups within your local churches, temples, or synagogues, or other places of worship that cater to your particular faith tradition (e.g., Christianity, Catholicism, Judaism, etc.).

You can also enhance your practice with mindfulness tools like guided meditation apps, calming music, or mindfulness journals.

In addition to these tools, explore the many mindfulness apps and online platforms available. Apps like Headspace, Calm, and Insight Timer offer guided meditations, exercises, and progress tracking to support your practice. Online platforms often provide courses, community forums, and live events, creating a comprehensive mindfulness experience. When choosing apps and platforms, consider your needs and preferences, look for reputable and well-reviewed options, and check for senior-friendly features and accessibility.

And finally, you can also explore various online communities and platforms dedicated to mindfulness, where you can connect with others and access a wealth of resources.

VII. Following Your Inner Compass—Shaping Your Journey:

As you've journeyed through these pages, I've presented the idea that mindfulness does not have to be a rigid practice incorporating rules, specific goals, and ideal outcomes, but rather, a flexible Life Tool for navigating life's joys, sorrows, and complexities. You've been invited to listen to and honor your inner compass, that quiet voice of intuition that supports your joy and well-being. Trust in your ability to shape, adapt, and adjust your own path, using the tools and strategies we've outlined to create a mindfulness approach that resonates with your unique needs and aspirations.

Remember, your journey is your own, and you now possess many resources to chart a wisdom-driven course to support you and your life.

But let's not forget that like any journey, mindfulness may present you with a variety of challenges. You may find it difficult to maintain consistency, experience moments of frustration or doubt, or lose motivation or momentum. These experiences are a natural part of the process. We hope that the resources we've outlined will encourage and support you on your journey.

In the end, from my perspective, mindfulness is not about achieving perfection, but rather revealing it, not about cultivating awareness and compassion, but rather, settling into awareness and allowing compassion to naturally arise.

Be patient with yourself, and celebrate all the forward and backward steps, as they are your guideposts for your journey ahead. If you find yourself struggling, revisit the core principles we have outlined in the first chapters of the book (Chapters 1 through 4) that include the essential foundational concepts and exercises that will never lead you astray. And remember, with one single mindful breath, you can drop into the power of the present moment where your potential for renewal and new beginnings lies.

VIII. Final Thoughts and Encouragement:

As we reach the end of our shared exploration, I want to leave you with a final thought: Your mindfulness adventure is just beginning. Embrace the journey in the gentle spirit of curious self-inquiry, and embrace your own naturally revealed compassion for yourself and others. Each moment offers an opportunity to pivot, transform, and embody your highest self. The benefits of continued engagement with mindfulness are immeasurable. So, step forward with confidence, knowing that you have the tools to navigate life's ever-shifting landscape with a natural grace and inherent resilience that will carry you forward into new adventures and joys.

BACK MATTER TABLE OF CONTENTS

About the Author

Hello, I am Blair O'Neil, a 50+ year
mindfulness advocate and practitioner,
and the author and founder of
Mindfulness for Seniors.

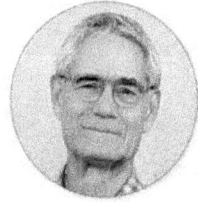

As for my journey into mindfulness:

It actually started as a senior in High School (1972) in the
vibrant and diverse beach scene of Southern California.
Growing up in Santa Monica and Venice, my life was shaped
by chance encounters with artists, beach musicians, surfers,
spiritual teachers, and the rich and colorful tapestry of the
diverse local community. That mixed with the soothing
and familiar smell of the ocean, the intoxicating rhythmic
beat of conga drummers, and the continual ebb and flow
of the pulsing waves, juxtaposed against a backdrop of
stark contrasts where creative expressions of humanity
mingled and mixed with lives full of sorrow and struggle,
all contributed to the formative experience that still brings
joy and gratitude to my heart. Over the years and through
many seemingly unrelated coincidences, mishaps, joys, and
sorrows, my explorations of various spiritual traditions,
some of which incorporated mindfulness approaches,
eventually led me to more formal training in Buddhism,
Vajrayana, and eventually, Dzogchen.

In this book, I have shared the insights and practices that
have been most helpful to me in navigating the challenges

and joys of life, including those from my formative years and the decades that followed, extending now into my senior years.

My aim has been to offer a "distilled and essential version" of what helped me, incorporating a friendly, gentle, practical, and easy-to-use approach to mindfulness, free from the barriers and obstacles of jargon, rigor, and prescriptive methods that are so commonly encountered in mindfulness teachings, which made up a large part of my own journey.

In these pages, I hope readers will benefit from my words of encouragement and support and find value in the tools and insights that have been shared, all intended to add some sense of comfort and ease while aiding you in reclaiming your own natural joy.

If you would like to learn more about me, please visit: mindfulness4seniors.com/about

Or use the QR code below:

Or Connect & Follow On:

YouTube:
youtube.com/@MindfulnessForSeniors

Facebook:
facebook.com/MindfulnessForSeniors

Web: mindfulness4seniors.com

Further Support & Resources

1) Mindfulness Resources for Seniors and their Caregivers: Explore the free curated collection of accessible mindfulness resources designed to support your well-being and mindfulness journey. Discover guided meditations, gentle exercises, informative articles, and recommended apps tailored for seniors, pre and post menopausal women, and those navigating the empty nest. Find practical tools and information to enhance your journey towards greater ease, emotional and mental calm, and finding joy.

Access at: tinyurl.com/Resources-for-Seniors

Or use the QR Code below:

Mindfulness Resources for Seniors, Menopausal Women, and Empty Nesters

Practical tools and information to enhance your well-being through mindfulness.

In addition to our book, 'Mindfulness for Seniors-A Flexible Wisdom-Driven Approach for Revealing Joy & Meeting Life's Challenges,' and our companion '100 Mindful Moments for Seniors: Savoring Life,' we've gathered a variety of additional easy-to-use resources, that include guided meditations, gentle exercises, informative articles, and recommended apps, all designed to support you on your mindfulness journey. These resources were chosen to support seniors, and help make mindfulness practical and enjoyable. We hope you find the following resources helpful.

2) "Inspired by Joy" Newsletter:

Receive my free bi-weekly mindfulness inspiration newsletter designed to support your journey towards greater well-being. Join our community for gentle guidance, practical tips, uplifting stories, and updates on events, podcasts, and new resources, all tailored to the unique experiences of seniors.

Learn More at: tinyurl.com/Newsletter-Information

Or use the QR Code below:

Inspired by Joy

Mindfulness For Seniors

Top stories from the community

Our "Inspired by Joy" Newsletter sends bi-weekly mindfulness inspiration designed to support your journey towards greater well-being. Join our community for gentle guidance, practical tips, uplifting stories, and updates on events, podcasts, and new resources, all tailored to the unique experiences of seniors

3) Senior-Only Free Online Community:

Join the waiting list to be part of this vibrant, inclusive community when it launches. This founder-led private online forum is designed to be a supportive and jargon-free space exclusively for seniors seeking a shared mindfulness connection.

Learn More: tinyurl.com/Senior-Only-Community

Or use the QR Code below:

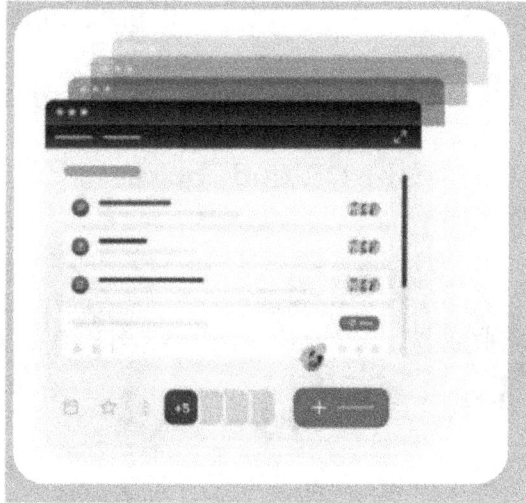

4) 100 Mindful Moments for Seniors: Introducing *"100 Mindful Moments for Seniors: Savoring Life,"* a collection of joyful, easy-to-use, and budget-friendly exercises exploring the richness of sensory mindfulness. This companion book offers 100 unique and practical ways to engage your senses and cultivate a deeper appreciation for each moment, complementing the broader wisdom offered in the overview book, "Mindfulness for Seniors." Inside, you'll find 100 easy, safe, fun, and enjoyable mindfulness exercises (20 per sense), organized by the five senses: sight, sound, smell, taste, and touch.

Learn More at: tinyurl.com/100-Mindful-Moments

Or use the QR Code below:

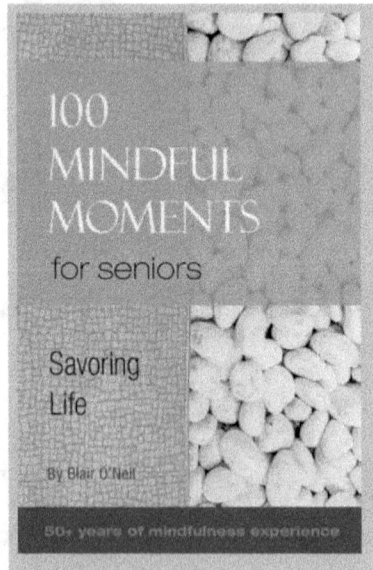

100
MINDFUL
MOMENTS
for seniors

Savoring
Life

By Blair O'Neil

50+ years of mindfulness experience

5) For Professionals & Organizations: Blair O'Neil also works with senior care organizations, medical and mental health professionals and practices, as well as businesses to help them integrate the practical, wisdom-driven principles from this book. To learn more about custom workshops, staff resilience programs, or strategic consulting, please visit:

Learn More at: mindfulness4seniors.com/services

Or use this QR Code:

Appendix A:

An Effective Calming Tool
for Intense Emotions

(This approach is inspired by concepts from Dialectical Behavior Therapy. See the "For Further Reading" section at the end of this appendix for more information.)

What it is: A Simple Tool to Cool the Flames of Upset

There are moments when an emotional storm can feel all-consuming, making it difficult to find your footing. *(See Chapter 7, pages 173 to 178, for other approaches to help with intense emotional storms.)* When mindfulness feels out of reach and an upset has taken over, this simple and powerful tool can be your anchor. Think of it as a life preserver tossed to you in turbulent waters. By gently shifting your attention to the world around you, you can steady yourself and reconnect to your natural ease.

Why This Is a Powerful "Upset Interrupt"

When we're caught in an emotional upset, our mind can feel like a runaway train, gathering speed with distressing thoughts and feelings. This tool acts as a reliable, effective, and gentle "reset button." Let's be clear, it doesn't erase the reason for the upset, but it does interrupt its overwhelming momentum. It helps prevent us from saying or doing things we might later regret—protecting our relationships and our own sense of well-being. By giving your mind a new focus, you create a small buffer of space. In that buffer, you can catch your breath, regain your mental and emotional balance, and eventually choose how to respond, rather than being carried away by the storm.

How It Works: Giving Your Mind an Easy Job

An upset mind is trying to do a very hard job with no instructions. This tool works by giving your mind a new, and very easy, job to do. Instead of trying to "fix" the difficult feeling(s), you simply ask your mind to do something else that is easy, like "notice things that are green" or "count the pictures on the wall." This simple act shifts your brain's focus and response away from the upset and upheaval toward a calmer, receptive state that can more easily navigate the challenge. It's a very effective way to signal to your nervous system that it's okay to stand down from high alert. And remember, we aren't getting rid of the feelings; we're just turning down the heat so we can handle them with a bit more ease and grace.

When and How to Use This Effective & Flexible Tool

This tool is especially helpful when you feel too overwhelmed for other calming approaches. It's a first step back to solid ground. In the Mindfulness for Seniors phrasing, we simply refer to this as the "Just Notice 10 Things" Strategy. On the next page are some examples.

• **Try Counting:** Casually count "just 10 things" around you. It could be ten books on a shelf or ten leaves on a plant. The number isn't as important as the gentle act of looking and counting.

• **Try Naming Colors:** Look around you and silently name five things you can see that are green. Then four things that are brown. Then three things that are yellow. Repeat as needed with any colors you see.

• **Try Noticing Textures:** Without moving, notice the feeling of your feet on the floor. Or reach out and touch the fabric of your chair. Focus all your attention on that single sensation for a moment.

Remember, this is your tool. We encourage you to make it your own. If counting 'ten things' isn't enough, count to twenty. If focusing on colors works better for you than textures, do that. The only rule is this: If it helps you regain your natural calm, it is the right way to use the tool.

For Further Reading

The core of this strategic life tool and technique is adapted from well-researched therapeutic approaches, most notably Dialectical Behavior Therapy (DBT). For those interested in the clinical background of these kinds of techniques, searching online for "DBT Distress Tolerance Skills" will provide a wealth of information.

Index of Key Concepts

Index of Key Concepts

Index Continues Next Page...

Index of Key Concepts

Index Continues Next Page...